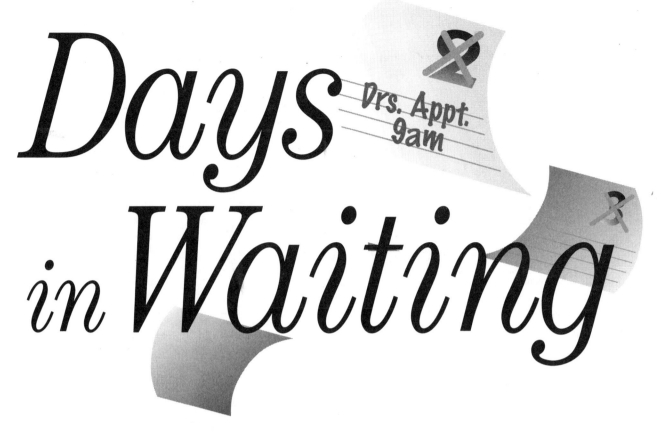

Days in Waiting

A Guide to Surviving Pregnancy Bedrest

by Mary Ann McCann

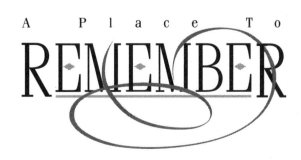

A Place To REMEMBER

A Subsidiary of deRuyter-Nelson Publications, Inc.
Saint Paul, Minnesota

DAYS IN WAITING
A GUIDE TO SURVIVING PREGNANCY BEDREST

Cover Design by Bob Wasiluk

Publication Data
McCann, Mary Ann

Printed in the United States of America

deRuyter-Nelson Publications, Inc.
1885 University Avenue, Suite 110
Saint Paul, Minnesota 55104

Table Of Contents:

Pregnancy is supposed to be one of the happiest times in a woman's life. The miracle of life is an awesome gift. For most women, pregnancy is a time to reflect, prepare, and anticipate all that a new child will bring to her life, as well as that of her husband or partner, other children, and extended family.

For some women, a joyful, miraculous pregnancy can suddenly become one of the greatest challenges she'll ever face. When complications arise, women are often sent to bed, either on modified or total bedrest. This can be a startling development that disrupts every aspect of her and her family's life.

My book is intended to present some of the many issues that a woman on bedrest may face. I hope the workbook format, with checklists and space for recording answers to the questions you will have for your doctor, will make this book a useful tool as well as source of support. Although I make numerous references to my own diagnoses, conditions, and treatments, the book is not intended to serve as a medical reference or substitute for proper medical attention. Each woman, and each pregnancy, is unique. My experiences and treatments may or may not be similar.

It is my hope that what I have written will give women on bedrest inspiration to cope with the daily challenges of a difficult pregnancy and commend them for their spirit and strength.

I owe a debt of gratitude to the many people who inspired me and encouraged me to write this book.

The staff of the United Hospital Birth Center, where I received most of my prenatal and antepartal care, are some of the most committed and dedicated individuals I have had the pleasure of knowing. I thank them for their compassion and encouragement.

I wish to thank Annette Klein, Carolyn Spenser, Jessie Tomlin, Tonia Smith, Pat Schaffner, and Dr. Tom Grande for reading my chapters, offering their advice and sharing their knowledge.

I am eternally grateful to the many bedrest mothers who honestly and openly shared their stories with me and offered me new insights. I would like to thank Shirley Audorff, Jessie Tomlin, and Valeri Gore for sharing their experiences of raising children while on bedrest. Their ideas and suggestions are incorporated into Chapter 7.

Thank you to my family and friends, especially the women in my Encountering Couples group who continued to support and encourage this endeavor. Your interest in my efforts and progress were a great inspiration.

Finally, it is with deep love and gratitude that I dedicate this book to my loving, supportive husband, Kelly, and to my own little miracles, William John and Colin James. You each bring love, joy, and purpose to every day.

Mary Ann McCann

One Woman's Story

I was on extended bedrest during both of my pregnancies, so I have little knowledge of worry-free, normal pregnancy. I envied women who were able to work, care for their families, take care of their homes, shop, prepare for a new baby, and enjoy a normal relationship with their husbands. But while the losses were real, there were positive things as well.

I survived two difficult pregnancies to be the proud mother of two beautiful, healthy little boys. While I would not wish my difficult experiences on anyone, I have come to value the lessons that I  learned about myself. I am a stronger, more patient and accepting person than I was before. The same is true for my husband, Kelly. And I am proud to say that my marriage is stronger for the struggles that we shared. We worked hard to bring our boys into the world, and we will never take them for granted, nor will we ever cease to be amazed and grateful for the love and joy that they bring to our lives.

When I was 12 weeks pregnant with our first child, Kelly and I enjoyed a romantic four-day weekend on the shore of Lake Superior in northern Minnesota. It was autumn, and a beautiful time to enjoy the woods and water. We relaxed and had a glorious time, realizing this would be our last chance to get away, alone, before our baby arrived. On the way home I felt a pain on the right side of my abdomen. At first I thought it was nothing. As we drove, the pain increased and I told Kelly that I was afraid something was wrong. As soon as we arrived home I called my OB/GYN's office and spoke to the on-call doctor. He told me to come to the office as soon as they opened in the morning. I was filled with a fear I had never felt before.

The next day I saw my doctor and he ordered an ultrasound. Kelly met me at the hospital and we waited for what seemed like an eternity. I was so nervous and scared. The ultrasound showed that I had a placental abruption, which meant that the placenta was starting to pull away from the wall of the uterus. I was told to stay in bed until my condition stabilized. I called work and told my boss that I wasn't sure when I would be returning, but that I hoped it wouldn't be longer than a week.

Within a matter of days I started bleeding. My doctor then told me that I would have to stay on total bedrest. He said he wanted to see me more frequently, and was especially fond of the saying, "Let's just see where things are at next week." I had to learn to live day to day and week to week.

At about 16 weeks I started having contractions and was diagnosed with pre-term labor. I realized I would not be returning to work until after my baby was born. It was a difficult thing to accept because I loved my job and was already bored being confined to bed. It seemed like the pregnancy would last forever. My doctor wanted me to continue carrying this baby as long as possible and told me to concentrate on the goal of making it to at least 28 weeks. I had to face reality – ten more weeks of total bedrest. "I can do it," I thought.

I was given oral Terbutaline along with Vistaril for the side effects, which included a racing pulse and shortness of breath. As the weeks progressed, my frequency and intensity of contractions increased. By

Christmas I was taking two Terbutaline tablets every two hours, and yet I was still contracting as often as every 6-8 minutes. I was shaky and so short of breath from the Terbutaline that I could no longer have a five-minute telephone conversation without panting and feeling like I had just run a marathon.

At 28 weeks I was hospitalized. The contraction activity was steadily increasing and the oral Terbutaline was becoming less effective. I was "loaded" on Magnesium Sulfate to quiet my overactive uterus. My first 48 hours of Magnesium Sulfate are still a blur. I have vague recollections of family members coming to visit me, although I don't remember conversations. I felt tired, nauseated, and drunk. I had blurry vision and little control over my muscles. I needed assistance to use the bathroom because I couldn't feel my legs. I will never forget having to buzz for a nurse to come and help me cut my breakfast of scrambled eggs and pancakes. I finally called Kelly and sobbed. As my uterus quieted, I was gradually titrated down from the high levels of Magnesium Sulfate and began to feel a bit more like myself.

Within 72 hours of admission, I was started on a Terbutaline sub-cutaneous (under the skin) pump. This was a miracle for me, as it is for many women. The Terbutaline is released continuously throughout the body, giving some relief from the terrible side effects. I was taught how to prepare a site, which is most often in the thigh. Although I was worried that I would have difficulty poking a needle and tube into my leg, it was surprisingly easy. Medical staff taught me how to program the little computerized box which held the small syringe of liquid Terbutaline. The syringe was screwed into a thin three foot tube that went directly into my upper thigh. I was taught how to change the syringes (two times each day) and how to change a site (every two to three days, alternating thighs). As the Terbutaline pump started to work, I was further titrated off of the Magnesium Sulfate, until I was completely off.

My doctors also started me on bi-weekly intra-muscular injections of Betamethasone, a steroid that accelerates the development of the baby's lungs. The first injection was given at the hospital, but a nurse had to show Kelly how to prepare and administer the rest of the injections, which he gave me in the buttocks.

After a couple more days of adjusting my pump dosages, I was released. The last stop on our way out of the hospital was to the Neonatal Intensive Care Unit (NICU) – a routine tour for women in high-risk pregnancies. While it is difficult to face the possibility of giving birth to a premature baby, it can be helpful for parents to have an opportunity to see the unit. Kelly and I were shocked to see tiny babies, many weighing less than three pounds, hooked up to monitors, ventilators, and I.V. pumps. The nurses explained what the various machines and monitors were for. The final stop was to the incubator of a 28-week baby so we would appreciate just how small our baby would be if he were born this early. We were both scared. I will never forget the image of that tiny little girl. Her father was next to the incubator reading her a Dr. Seuss story. I felt a lump in my throat and tears burning my eyes. I looked up at Kelly – he, too, had tears. During our ride home we talked about our renewed commitment to doing everything possible to keep our baby inside of me as long as possible.

The Terbutaline pump made life a lot easier and I also received in-home health care from a nurse two or three times each week. The visits included time on a fetal monitor, which I enjoyed, since it gave me the opportunity to hear my baby's heartbeat. The nurse looked at my records of contraction activity, and, if necessary, helped me make changes in the pump dosages. She also performed some routine blood and urine tests. Because I was so lonely, I looked forward to the home visits.

I continued to see my doctor once a week and looked forward to those appointments. Kelly also enjoyed the doctor visits and took time off from work to accompany me. We loved watching the movements of our little boy on the ultrasound. The nurse took measurements and I liked knowing how much he had grown in the past week. That was an essential motivator for me – I could feel pride in accomplishing another week of growth for the baby. My doctor was understanding of my increasing levels of stress and exhaustion and kept telling me to think about making it to week 32.

Week 32 came and went. Naturally, I expected some answers and direction from my doctor, but he decided my new goal was week 34. While I knew that was the best thing for the baby, I fell apart and sobbed in his office. Kelly looked at him and said, "She's been in bed for 20 weeks. I'm not sure how much more of this she can handle." The doctor was sympathetic but asked us to continue on for the sake of our son. I knew he was right, but still I cried all the way home.

For a couple of days I was very depressed. I was on higher levels of Terbutaline and still contracting at least every eight minutes. The contractions were becoming harder, sharper, and lasting longer. Because of the contractions, I was unable to sleep through the night and I worried about how they were affecting the baby. Whenever I had the sharp, painful contractions, the baby kicked or punched back.

It was about this time I began to finally realize that I was going to have this baby. The realization seemed crazy – after all, I had been in bed for 20 weeks thinking about little else. But I had been completely focused on *not* having the baby, and now the time had finally come to prepare for his arrival.

I became very depressed. I couldn't have a baby shower (my sister had already planned to give me a shower after the baby was born), I couldn't attend childbirth classes, and I wasn't able to do any of my own shopping.

Kelly went shopping and purchased layette clothing, hooded towels, washcloths, snap shirts, and terry snapsuits. He came home from the store so excited and proud of himself at what he had accomplished. All I could do was cry – I wanted to be the one to decide whether to buy sheets with polka dots or bears. I didn't realize then that I was feeling a normal loss. There were many losses to contend with and this was just one of many. Looking back, I realize that that was a significant moment for Kelly. He had spent much of the previous 20 weeks worried that we would lose this baby, so making those purchases was a way for him to put that fear behind him and focus on the future.

At 34 weeks, I had enough. My doctor performed an amniocentesis which showed that the baby's lungs were mature. I made the decision (with my doctor's approval) to pull the pump out of my leg for the last time. We were prepared to have the baby within 24 hours of discontinuing the Terbutaline. While my contractions became more frequent and painful, I did not go into hard labor.

On March 3, I was admitted to the hospital for labor induction. We chose to induce because my contraction activity, especially after the pump was discontinued, made my life a living hell. I contracted every three minutes, and the contractions often lasted 60 seconds. They were so sharp and hard I was no longer able to talk through them and many brought tears to my eyes. Because this was my first baby, it was expected that induction would be slow. But, I had lost patience. I had been patient for 22 weeks, and I just wanted that baby out. Unfortunately, the induction was slow and frustrating.

At about 10:00 a.m. March 4 my doctor broke my bag of waters, sending me into hard labor. I was thankful to receive an epidural at 11:00 a.m.. After so many weeks of contractions, I was grateful for some relief.

By 4:30 p.m. I was fully dilated. I pushed five times and the baby's head crowned. My doctor arrived at 5:10, and William John McCann entered the world at 5:15, weighing 5 pounds, 3 ounces. He was strong, had good color, and he was breathing on his own. Because he was a premature baby, there were three nurses from the NICU present for his birth. As soon as they heard his hardy cry, they knew they were no longer needed. William was immediately given to Kelly and me. I will never forget the feeling of gratitude and relief. After having spent so many weeks waiting and worrying, the feelings were overwhelming. William and I were discharged 48 hours later, and we were finally able to enjoy this beautiful baby we had worked so hard to bring into the world.

The Next Pregnancy

We loved William so much and decided that we really wanted to have another baby – for ourselves, as well as for him. We knew there was a chance that I could have another difficult pregnancy.

Unfortunately, I did not get pregnant as quickly as we hoped. I had been taking my temperature and soon realized that I was not ovulating. After an examination my doctor prescribed Clomid, a drug that induces ovulating. I started ovulating with my first cycle after starting the drug. I continued to take my morning temperatures, chart mucus, and time intercourse as carefully as possible.

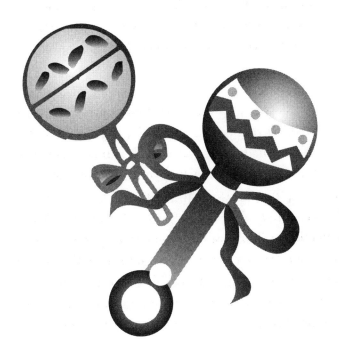

After eleven months, my doctor decided it was time to run some more diagnostic tests. I was scheduled for a Hysterosalpingogram (HSG) where the doctor injects dye through the cervix. The dye follows the uterus into and through the fallopian tubes. Although I did not have blockage in either of my tubes, it was discovered that I had a bicornet uterus. There was a muscle-like wall that started at the top of the uterus, and extended down about 75% of the way, offering an obvious explanation for my difficult pregnancy. The fertilized egg had implanted on one side of the wall (referred to as a horn), and the fetus had grown in just half of the uterus. Because half is not enough space, the uterine horn grew too large, and the contractions began.

The most stressful part of learning this was the knowledge that I would have another difficult pregnancy, possibly worse than the first. Kelly and I never wavered in our decision to have another baby, however, and we continued with our efforts to become pregnant. After having laproscopic surgery to clean scar tissue from the first pregnancy out of my uterus, I was finally able to get pregnant.

From the day that my home pregnancy test turned pink, I began a modified form of bedrest. I no longer lifted William (or anything else) and stopped performing most forms of housework. I quit substitute teaching. I laid on the couch for several hours a day. I really believed that a more sedate lifestyle would postpone the inevitable.

At approximately 11 weeks I started contracting. It was too soon to start Terbutaline, so I had to just concentrate on resting. I hired two college women to spend a few hours each morning with William so I could rest. William loved the extra attention and I was grateful for the opportunities he had to get outside and play.

At the end of March we had to enroll William in a full-time Montessori school because my doctor ordered strict bedrest. This was a tremendous stress as I worried more about how the pregnancy was going to effect William. He loved his new school and was always eager to go, but it was still difficult to spend my days in bed while he was in daycare.

Kelly was wonderful about taking on additional responsibilities. He never complained, and concentrated completely on the pregnancy, doing whatever he could to make things easier for me.

We lived 60 minutes away from the hospital and my doctor, and it soon became clear that we couldn't stay in Northfield for the entire pregnancy. We also knew that we couldn't continue to send William to Montessori because I was unable to drive him. So, at the beginning of June we moved into my mother-in-law's home. Joan was gracious and generous to offer her home to us and help us with William. Kelly's brother, Mike, lived across the street and his wife, Kadee, offered to care for William during the summer. William was ecstatic to spend the summer with his four cousins and we were happy that everything seemed to be working out so well.

Three days after we moved into Joan's home, I was hospitalized. My contractions were too strong and frequent, even with the Terbutaline. I expected that I would be in for a few days and start the Terbutaline pump, like I had with my first pregnancy. Unfortunately that did not work and I required intravenous Magnesium Sulfate to keep my contraction activity under control. Each time they attempted to wean me from the Magnesium, I contracted too much. They increased my

Terbutaline levels, but each time they decreased the Magnesium the results were the same – stronger, more frequent contractions. After two trials on the Terbutaline pump and three weeks of hospitalization, I faced the hard reality: I wasn't going home. Although Kelly and I both went through an initial denial phase, we soon found ourselves making preparations for me to spend the summer in the hospital.

Even though I was on high levels of Magnesium Sulfate, I was still contracting at least every 10 minutes. The evenings were the worst, since if I had more than six or seven contractions during the hour that I was on the monitor, I required Terbutaline shots. Most evenings I needed two or three shots to space the contractions out to 10-12 minutes apart. Unfortunately the shots were only given at 60-minute intervals, so many evenings I was on the monitor for three or four hours.

My greatest anxiety was over William's well-being. I knew that my mother-in-law and sister-in-law were caring for him and that Kelly was doing everything he could, but it wasn't enough. I missed Will terribly. Because he was just a little more than two, his speech limited our telephone conversations and he was quite bored in my hospital room when he made his daily visits. Luckily, he accepted the explanation that mommy needed to stay in the hospital to take care of the baby. Kelly often took him to the newborn nursery to show him the babies and we would talk about our baby coming out after he was done growing. William probably thought that our situation was normal; he knew of no other way for a mommy to have a baby.

The weeks dragged on. I began working with a group of specialists who performed biophysical profiles (a more detailed ultrasound) two to three times per week. I looked forward to this outing, even if it was only an elevator ride in a wheelchair. That's how mundane my life had become.

Despite my attempts to be positive and cheerful, I had many days of great sadness. I was pregnant with my second son (and that was all that mattered) but I never anticipated that I would spend so much time hospitalized on drugs that made me feel so sick. I received another anti-labor drug, Indocin, for about four weeks. The Indocin, in combination with the Magnesium Sulfate, brought me relief from the contractions, and I no longer required the Terbutaline shots every night. Unfortunately, Indocin can pose certain risks for a baby, particularly beyond the 32nd week of gestation. So after a small hiatus, I was back to contractions and Terbutaline shots. I also received Betamethasone injections (to accelerate the baby's lung development) for several weeks, which increased the frequency and severity of my migraines and caused vomiting.

The biophysical profiles started to show that I no longer had enough amniotic fluid in my uterus. Various possible explanations were given, but the only one I really heard was the worst possibility: kidney malformation or dysfunction in the baby. I had dreams at night of bringing my newborn into the hospital for dialysis. The fluid levels never again returned to normal. We were also told that our baby showed signs of IUGR, (intrauterine growth retardation) essentially meaning that the baby was growing too slowly. He was about two weeks behind, so my due date was actually changed to October 15 instead of September 30. That was not good news since it meant that I would have to be hospitalized even longer.

On August 16 I had an amniocentesis to check the baby's lung maturity. I was warned that the lungs might be too immature to even discuss the possibility of having the baby. Happily, the news turned out to be somewhat positive: the lungs were considered borderline, so the time was rapidly approaching for this baby to enter the world.

On August 22, exactly 11 weeks after I had first been admitted to the hospital, I was transferred to the Labor and Delivery Unit to begin labor induction. Because of my bicornet uterus, induction was difficult...I contracted every 90 seconds, but didn't dilate. After twelve hours on I.V. Pitosin, contracting every 90-120 seconds, all that had been accomplished was total effacement, softening of the cervix, and dilation to one. I was so depressed. I sobbed uncontrollably and saw my husband looking at me with worry. He knew I couldn't handle much more. To add to my problems, I had taken a bad fall that evening and broken my tailbone.

My doctor arrived at 6:30 the following morning promising results. Because I was dilated to one, he told me that he would attempt to

break my bag of waters. He believed that my body was too exhausted to endure a long labor, so breaking my water would speed things up. After several attempts, he said that he wasn't able to feel the baby's head and was concerned that the baby had rotated. He planned to stay in the hospital and monitor me. After a couple of hours, as the Pitosin increased the intensity of the contractions, the baby started going into distress, with his heart rate dropping drastically each time I contracted. My doctor turned me from one side to the other, trying to increase blood flow to the baby, but nothing helped. I was petrified! I watched my baby's heart rate drop from 135 beats/minute to 90, then 70, then 40, with each contraction.

The doctor decided to perform an emergency C-section. Within 30 minutes I was in the operating room receiving an epidural. After I was prepped for surgery, Kelly came in to be with me. As soon as the team from the Neonatal Intensive Care Unit (NICU) arrived, it was time to deliver. I was amazed at how quickly they worked. It was difficult for them to access the baby and they had to make additional incisions and spend several minutes pushing down on the top of my uterus.

At 10:35, Colin James McCann arrived. He was immediately taken to the NICU nurses and given oxygen. He was small and weak, but attempting to breathe on his own. They brought him over to me for a few minutes before they took him away. He was perfect. I couldn't believe that he was real. It seemed like the pregnancy had taken an eternity, and I felt an unbelievable sense of relief that it was finally over and he was okay. Colin weighed in at 4 pounds, 8 ounces, and only required minimal oxygen for the first 24 hours. He received light therapy for jaundice and was hooked up to an apnea monitor for several days.

Colin was released from the NICU on August 31, weighing just 3 pounds, 15½ ounces. Because we were not able to go back to Northfield for a couple more days, I took Colin to my parents' home and stayed with them. He needed to be awakened for feedings every 1½ -2 hours. I worried after every feeding – he never took as much as he was supposed to because he fell asleep soon after a feeding began.

I was exhausted, weak, and still in pain from the C-section, but I had my beautiful little boy and I was finally about to go home.

Chapter Two:

Bedrest: Words Of Acceptance

E ach year thousands of women are put on bedrest as a result of complications in their pregnancies. It is estimated that one out of every four pregnancies is considered high-risk. This is the equivalent of 800,000 - 1,000,000 women each year that face a high-risk pregnancy. Bedrest is the most common treatment for the varying problems associated with high-risk pregnancies.

Reasons For Bedrest

There are several reasons why a woman may be put on bedrest: multiple pregnancy, premature rupture of the membranes (also called the bag of waters), premature labor, pregnancy induced hypertension, problems with the placenta such as placental abruption, (a separation of the placenta from the uterine wall) placenta previa (placenta that slips down and partially or completely covers the cervix), and other pre-existing medical conditions, such as diabetes, Lupus, or high blood-pressure. Since this book is not intended to serve as a medical resource, I will not be offering any explanations of these conditions. If your doctor has ordered bedrest, you probably already know the reason.

You may have been told that your bedrest will be for a specific period of time, or your doctor may have told you that he/she is uncertain what the length of time will be. A multitude of pregnancy conditions require women to stay on bedrest for the duration of the pregnancy. Many doctors order bedrest until the 37th week of pregnancy. After that milestone has been reached (and it is a milestone), you may be able to increase your activity level until you deliver.

If your doctor tells you that he/she is uncertain about the duration of your bedrest, you will need to follow all orders carefully. This can be frustrating for women who have children at home to care for or a job outside the home.

With my first pregnancy, my doctor told me that he thought that I would be able to return, at least part-time, to my job. My employer waited for weekly updates about my condition. It was not until I began experiencing premature labor that my doctor was able to tell me that I would be spending the remainder of my pregnancy on bedrest.

Many women spend a few weeks on bedrest and are then able to return to a modified level of activity. Your cooperation and adherence to your doctor's recommendations are crucial.

You may be told that you will need to be on bedrest until your baby is born. This may mean anything from days, to weeks, to months. If you are told to stay in bed, you need to realize that your condition warrants it. Noncompliance with your doctor's orders could jeopardize your health and the health of your baby.

You will also be given information about how your doctor defines bedrest. Your doctor should be specific in his/her orders. If you are at all unclear about what level of activity you are able to participate in, it is important that you seek clarification. At the end of this chapter I have included some of the important questions you may need to ask your doctor. Your doctor may order modified bedrest or complete bedrest.

Modified Bedrest

If your doctor orders modified bedrest, this may mean that he/she will allow you to work part-time, if you are employed outside your home and if your job does not pose risks to the health of you or your baby. It could mean that your doctor does not want you working but will tolerate light household activity. Many doctors use the 50/10 rule: during each hour, you may engage in ten minutes of light activity, and then spend the next 50 minutes in bed. This form of bedrest often allows for the opportunity to perform light tasks around the house, or engage in activity with your family.

If your doctor orders modified bedrest, you must use great caution. You will have days when you feel good and will tell yourself that, "10 more minutes working in the kitchen won't hurt." It will be tempting to push yourself, especially when you are feeling well and concerned about the many responsibilities that are being neglected around the house.

When I was just nine weeks into my second bedrest, my doctor ordered modified bedrest. I admit that in the beginning I thought that modified bedrest meant that I should just rest when I was feeling tired or relax after the laundry was done. Kelly would come home from work to a hot meal on the table, a cake in the oven, folded clothes on the bed, and he would be upset with me for pushing myself. I would explain that I was feeling fine, and that I was not the slightest bit tired. He accompanied me to my next doctor visit and tattled about my lack of compliance. My doctor said something I will never forget. He asked me a crucial question: if I lost the baby tomorrow, would it be easier for me to accept the loss knowing that all the laundry was done and the bathroom was clean? I realized that I was risking the health of my baby in order to bake a cake. As difficult as it was, I complied with his orders.

Modified bedrest may be enough for you to successfully carry your baby to term without further complications. And modified bedrest may eventually allow you the opportunity to return to your job, family, and other responsibilities in a relatively short period of time. Or...you may be like the thousands of women who eventually end up on complete bedrest.

Complete Bedrest

Complete bedrest is exactly what it sounds like. For most doctors, complete bedrest means that you are allowed to get out of bed only for bathroom privileges, and in some cases, even bathroom trips are forbidden.

I often asked myself why using the toilet, something pregnant women do quite often, was suddenly a privilege?

Complete bedrest will probably mean that you will be expected to eat your meals in bed. In the most serious situations, you may be told to spend time laying on your right or left side only. Among other things, you may be restricted to showering every other day. Complete bedrest is a shock. You may go from full-time wife, mother, employee, homemaker, chauffeur, and chef, to pregnant woman on bedrest.

This is exactly how I felt when my doctor ordered complete bedrest with my first pregnancy. I think it took a little bit of time for it all to sink in. I asked a lot of questions, and didn't like the answers. "How about cooking?" "How about dusting the furniture or sweeping the floors?" "How about cleaning the bathroom?" "How about grocery shopping?" I admit I asked some pretty ridiculous questions. I think that I was just in a state of shock and denial. I guess I hoped that my doctor would answer yes to at least a couple of questions. It never happened – I received a resounding "no!" to each question. I eventually began to understand the magnitude of the situation. After I realized what I was expected to not do, I began the process of gradual acceptance.

Accepting Bedrest

Any form of bedrest is going to require a tremendous level of acceptance. You need to realize that bedrest may be the only way to ensure the health of you and your baby. There are so many medical cures and treatments available for people that it's easy to assume that a few pills or some new and advanced medical technology could be prescribed to eliminate bedrest. The truth is, there is nothing better than your own body to nurture your baby. Each day that you can carry this baby in your womb is truly a gift. You need to realize this if you are going to fully accept pregnancy bedrest. It may be a painful reality to accept, but you are nurturing your baby in the best way you can.

I spent a lot of days feeling depressed and inadequate because I thought there was something wrong with me. I knew so many women who had healthy pregnancies with no complications. For me, pregnancy is a large part of the experience of being a woman, and I wasn't able to do it right. I felt like less of a woman and that I was letting Kelly and myself down. When I was finally able to share my feelings with Kelly, it was the beginning of my journey to acceptance.

His support enabled me to feel okay about myself. Acceptance came gradually and I had to live one day at a time, reminding myself that each day of bedrest was a gift to my unborn child. Seeing the baby on the ultrasound screen and feeling him move were powerful reminders of what an important job I was fulfilling. Discovering the sex of each baby brought another level of commitment – we named each of our children and would often remind ourselves that every day was a gift for William and Colin.

Pregnancy complications can be mild, or they can be serious. Your doctor should fully describe the complications that you are facing, and what you should expect in the days and weeks ahead. It is critical that your partner be a part of your discussions with your doctor. If necessary, make an appointment to see your doctor as a couple or ask your doctor to arrange a phone conversation with your partner. Make sure that your partner understands the medical explanations given, as well as the recommendations regarding bedrest. It is crucial that you and your partner communicate openly and honestly during this time. You will both be facing many challenges and encountering emotions you've never shared before.

If your doctor tells you that your bedrest will be temporary, consider all of your doctor's bedrest recommendations carefully. Pushing your limits may ultimately increase the amount of time you will be on bedrest. You may want to ask your doctor how certain he/she is about the length of time they are estimating. If you are employed outside the home, your employer may need to make arrangements for your absence and will probably ask you if, when, and in what capacity, you will be returning to work.

Keep in mind that your situation could change tomorrow. Understanding the duration and level of your bedrest will also be crucial if you have other children, particularly if your are at home with them full-time. You will need to make childcare arrangements and your plans will have to be flexible as your pregnancy progresses.

If your doctor tells you that your bedrest is not temporary and that you need to be on bedrest until your baby is born, there will be a lot of important decisions to make. Again, it is critical that you and your partner be well informed about your medical condition and the exact level of bedrest required.

Below I have listed some of the concerns you and your partner may need to discuss. If you are spending your bedrest time in the hospital, many of these questions will be irrelevant and Chapter 4 will give you more information and suggestions about your hospitalization. As you read this list, jot down any additional questions you have and consider using a notebook where all your questions can be noted.

Children

What special plans do you need to make regarding your children – their current daycare/school arrangements, transportation arrangements, and other activities?

_____

_____

_____

_____

_____

_____

Are you able to care for your children by yourself?

_____

_____

_____

Can you arrange part-time help within your home, or will you need to arrange for full-time or part-time childcare?

_____

_____

_____

_____

What should you tell the children about mom's bedrest? Are they old enough to understand the situation without becoming too fearful?

_____

_____

_____

_____

Outside Employment

Contact your employer immediately and be honest about your situation. If you do not already know about the long-term and short-term disability benefits your employer offers, ask for a copy of the policy.

_____

_____

_____

_____

_____

Will your employer allow you to use unclaimed sick/vacation hours to apply to the disability-waiting period?

_____

_____

_____

_____

Is there an option for you to work part-time if your situation improves?

_____

_____

_____

_____

Is there an option for you to work on special projects or other responsibilities from your bed? (You need to talk with your doctor about whether this is allowed in your situation.)

_____

_____

_____

_____

If you receive medical insurance through your employer, you need to inquire immediately about how a short-term or long-term disability will affect your health coverage. You may need to begin paying part, or a larger part, of the premiums.

_____

_____

_____

_____

_____

_____

Finances

How will several days/weeks/months of bedrest affect you financially?

_____

_____

_____

_____

_____

_____

_____

Will there be a reduction in your monthly income? How much of a reduction? For how long?

_____

_____

_____

_____

_____

How will you pay for new expenses, such as medical costs, additional insurance costs, and additional daycare expenses?

_____

_____

_____

_____

_____

What sacrifices can you make to alleviate some of the financial burdens (cooking rather than ordering out, abstaining from use of credit cards, reducing the amount of money spent on gifts at holidays, etc.)? If your financial situation is going to be a tremendous burden, you may need to consider additional options, such as a second mortgage, loan consolidation or refinancing, loans from your family, or having your partner consider taking a second job during evenings and/or weekends.

_____

_____

_____

_____

_____

What plans do you need to make regarding the cleaning, cooking, shopping, yardwork, errands, and laundry responsibilities?

_____

_____

_____

_____

_____

_____

If applicable, what additional responsibilities can your children assume?

_____

_____

_____

_____

_____

_____

Can you afford to hire help for the housecleaning or yardwork?

_____

_____

_____

_____

_____

_____

Do you have friends or family willing to help with specific household responsibilities? If you have people willing to help, you might try to organize a schedule or chart, (i.e., asking a friend to come every Friday morning to clean in your kitchen, for example. Other friends or family members may be willing to come one evening per week to help with shopping or laundry.)

_____

_____

_____

_____

_____

_____

_____

_____

What responsibilities can you do from the confines of your bed (i.e., grocery lists, folding the laundry, paying the bills, balancing the checkbook, etc.)?

_____

_____

_____

_____

_____

_____

_____

_____

What other resources do you have to help – family, friends, church/temple communities, and your extended community?

_____

_____

_____

_____

_____

Personal Concerns

How do you want to explain your condition to your family and friends?

_____

_____

_____

_____

How can you and your partner arrange for personal time?

_____

_____

_____

_____

How much vacation/sick time does your partner have? How could you best utilize this time off? (Now or after the baby is born?)

_____

_____

_____

_____

Can you afford for your partner to take some Family Leave time? (There is a National Family Leave law requiring employers with more than 50 employees to give Family Leave time during a family emergency, or due to family illness.) Is it possible for your partner to work from home during part of the day? (This could be helpful if you have children.)

_____

_____

_____

_____

Additional Thoughts

_____

_____

_____

_____

_____

_____

_____

This list is just a starting point. You will be able to determine your own issues and needs after the reality of your condition sinks in. The following chapters will also help you and your partner cope with the difficulties of extended bedrest. You will have to keep reminding yourself of your goal. This bedrest will not last forever. You will survive, and, if you are like me, you will have a renewed perspective on life and a new sense of your strength as a woman.

Understanding Your Limitations

If you are on modified bedrest, the following is a list of questions you may want to ask your doctor. You will notice that I include a question pertaining to how each recommendation may change as your pregnancy progresses. You should attempt to gain a clear perspective about the outlook for the remainder of your pregnancy, especially if your doctor is prescribing bedrest during the second trimester. However, you should also be prepared for your doctor to tell you that he/she is uncertain how your condition will improve or worsen. It depends upon the specific complication(s), severity, and stage of pregnancy you are in. It may also depend upon your individual doctor. I know of women in situations similar to mine who were given more lenient orders. Because my doctor was conservative and cautious, I was on complete bedrest.

General Activity Level

How many minutes per hour (or every two or three hours, if necessary) can I engage in routine activity? 0? 10? 15? 20? How many minutes per hour do I need to be resting in bed? What position do I need to be in while I am in bed? (Your doctor may allow you to merely lie down, or he/she may tell you that you need to be on your left side. You may also need to elevate the foot of your bed.)

_____

_____

_____

_____

_____

_____

Is this recommendation likely to change as my pregnancy progresses? How might it change?

_____

_____

_____

_____

_____

May I continue to work at my current job, in my current position, in any capacity? (You may need to detail your job and your specific job responsibilities in order for him/her to adequately determine whether you may continue.)

_____

_____

_____

_____

_____

Is this recommendation likely to change as my pregnancy progresses? If yes, how might it change?

_____

_____

_____

_____

_____

Maintaining Your Home

Which of the following activities can I participate in? For what length of time? Are these recommendations and limitations likely to change as my pregnancy progresses? How might they change?

YES   NO

____   ____   Dusting – bending and reaching

_____

____   ____   Vacuuming – being on your feet, moving objects

_____

YES	NO	
___	___	Sweeping floors - some bending
___	___	Mopping/scrubbing floors - often on hands/knees
___	___	Cleaning bathroom - bending, strenuous scrubbing
___	___	Cooking - standing for long periods, bending, reaching
___	___	Laundry - bending, lifting, carrying
___	___	Mowing grass - strenuous pushing, may involve hills
___	___	Shoveling snow - bending, lifting, throwing
___	___	Raking leaves - bending, strenuous arm movements
___	___	Gardening - bending, reaching
___	___	Making/changing beds - bending and lifting the mattress
___	___	Ironing - standing for extended periods

Days in Waiting: *A Guide to Surviving Pregnancy Bedrest*

YES	NO	
___	___	Painting/decorating the nursery – standing, reaching

_____

YES	NO	
___	___	Washing dishes, loading or unloading dishwasher

_____

YES	NO	
___	___	Setting and clearing the dinner table

_____

Activities Outside Of Your Home

Which of the following outside activities may I participate in? For what length of time? Are these recommendations and limitations likely to change as my pregnancy progresses? How might they change? You should also ask your doctor if you are allowed to participate in any of these activities alone. Your doctor may not wish for you to be out by yourself, in the event of an emergency. This may be especially true for women in pre-term labor.

YES	NO	
___	___	Driving a car

_____

YES	NO	
___	___	Grocery shopping

_____

YES	NO	
___	___	Shopping for necessary baby items

_____

YES	NO	
___	___	Going to a movie, play, or concert

_____

YES	NO	
___	___	Going to a friend's home for the evening

_____

| ___ | ___ | Going to church/place of worship |

_____

| ___ | ___ | Participating in sporting activities (i.e., golf, swimming, aerobics, or other activities you routinely participate in) |

_____

| ___ | ___ | Going for a walk |

_____

Ask about any other pertinent activities you and your partner engage in.

_____

_____

_____

_____

_____

_____

_____

You may also need to clarify what your doctor will permit if your bedrest falls over a major holiday, such as Thanksgiving or Christmas, particularly if you had planned to travel.

Childcare

If you are an at-home mother, you will need to be clear about which, if any, of the routine aspects of childcare your doctor will allow you to participate in. If you are home with young toddlers or preschoolers this will be especially important to know. If your doctor orders modified bedrest, ask him/her to tell you what your specific limitations are, with respect to caring for your children, so that you and your partner can make proper arrangements.

YES   NO

___   ___   May I continue to care for my children as usual?

_____

_____

_____

___   ___   May I continue to lift my children? (This is a important consideration if you have toddlers.)

_____

_____

_____

___   ___   May I engage in playtime with my children, either inside or outside of the house? (You need to be clear about what activities are allowed, such as running.)

_____

_____

_____

_____

_____

_____

_____

___   ___   May I continue to bathe my children?

_____

_____

YES   NO

____   ____   Are these recommendations and limitations likely to change as my pregnancy progresses? How might they change?

_____

_____

_____

_____

Sexual Activity

This may be an uncomfortable issue to discuss with your doctor, but it is important for you to be clear about what you can and cannot participate in, particularly if your bedrest is going to be several months in duration. While your doctor may tell you that you should abstain from intercourse, many couples are able to explore new ways of sexually relating to each other once they are clear about their boundaries.

YES   NO

____   ____   May I engage in sexual activity that causes female orgasm?

_____

_____

_____

____   ____   May I engage in sexual activity that causes female arousal and stimulation?

_____

_____

_____

____   ____   May I engage in sexual intercourse? How often?

_____

YES   NO

___   ___   How will this change as my pregnancy progresses? Will I eventually have to abstain from all sexual activity?

_____

_____

_____

_____

_____

Other Considerations For Women On Complete, Long-term Bedrest

YES   NO

___   ___   May I use the bathroom regularly?

_____

_____

___   ___   Should I bathe or take a shower? How often?

_____

_____

___   ___   May I wash my hair? How often?

_____

_____

___   ___   Can I bathe, shower, or wash my hair if I use a bath seat? (Bath seats are available from medical supply companies, and some large drugstores. There are also companies that rent medical equipment.)

_____

_____

_____

_____

YES   NO

_____   _____   Can I eat my meals at the table, or do I need to eat in bed? Do I need to eat while lying in bed, or can I sit up with my back and neck supported?

_____

_____

_____   _____   Can I prepare simple meals for myself? (i.e., sandwiches, soup, salads, etc.)

_____

_____

When Can Activity Levels Increase?

_____

_____

_____

_____

_____

_____

_____

_____

It is perfectly normal if these questions cause some concern and worry. Remember, you will survive this. It will be easier to accept your bedrest once you are clear about the severity and limitations of your condition. The remainder of this book is dedicated to helping you cope with bedrest in the best possible way. Keep focusing on the fact that every day you are one-step closer to your goal...a healthy baby.

Chapter Three

Surviving Bedrest While At Home

Depending on the nature of your pregnancy complications, you may spend your time on bedrest at home. As I discussed in Chapter 2, it is important for you to have clear guidelines regarding your bedrest and the limitations that your doctor has given. If you are at all unclear whether a particular activity or household task is safe for you and your baby, contact your doctor's office before engaging in the activity. Nurses and nurse practitioners are often able to consult with patients regarding their bedrest restrictions. If you and your partner have looked at the questions I included in Chapter 2, you are probably already aware of your boundaries and limitations. This chapter is intended to offer some ideas for utilizing your time while in bed. Again, I cannot stress enough the importance of following your doctor's orders.

The Bedrest Environment

If your doctor orders modified bedrest, you will be spending several hours per day in bed. If your doctor has ordered complete bedrest, I hope that this chapter will give you some help in scheduling and planning your days. Take heart, there are plenty of things that you can do, even while you are in bed. If you read about a particular activity, and it causes you some concern, please call and ask whether you are able to participate in the activity in question. Each pregnancy is different, as is each doctor. Because I spent 22 weeks on complete bedrest with my first pregnancy, I can sympathize with those of you who are wondering how you will ever survive without going completely crazy. As the days, weeks and months progressed, I discovered new ideas for utilizing my time, and these helped me to combat boredom and depression. The place to begin, however, is analyzing your environment and making it conducive to bedrest.

Choosing The Best Bedrest Space

Whether your bedrest is temporary or lasting the duration of your pregnancy, it is important for you and your partner to spend some time planning for your needs.

You will probably be most comfortable in your own bed. As your pregnancy progresses, you will find yourself taking short naps. However, it may be that another part of your home will be a better place for you, particularly if you are not able to climb stairs. If it is possible, you may wish to equip two different locations, particularly if you know that you are going to be on bedrest for several weeks. If you have children, you may want one bedrest location conducive to short periods of game playing or story time.

There are several important questions to ask yourself before you determine where your bedrest space will be. You and your partner should discuss these questions before making your decision. Any time you spend planning and organizing your bedrest space will be time well spent.

Questions To Consider

1. Will your doctor permit you to climb stairs? If yes, do you need to limit the number of times per day that I use the stairs? How will this affect your decision about where to spend your bedrest?

2. How close is the nearest bathroom? Do you need to climb stairs to get to the bathroom?

3. Is there a telephone or telephone jack nearby? (Ideally, you should have a telephone next to you at all times.) Should you consider a portable phone?

4. How close is the kitchen? (This may not be an issue if your doctor is not permitting you to prepare your own meals.)

5. If you cannot prepare your own meals, what arrangements need to be made? (For example, can you arrange to have a cooler or dorm-sized refrigerator nearby?)

6. Would you like to have a television within viewing range? (They help to pass the time.) What about a VCR for viewing movies and tapes?

7. What type of table or bed trays do you have available to keep necessary items at close reach? Some of the many items you may need include:

- medications
- a thermos of ice water and a glass
- snacks (granola bars, crackers, cereal, etc.)
- pens and pencils
- writing paper
- address book, complete with your doctors' phone numbers
- art and craft supplies
- reading materials
- television program guides
- television and VCR remote controls
- lotion and lip balm

_____

_____

_____

_____

_____

As your bedrest progresses, you will keep adding necessities to your bed table. For example, I had a candy jar and my attentive husband took full responsibility for keeping it filled!

8. Would you like to have a stereo system nearby? If this is not possible, how about a Walkman-type system?

9. If your bedrest will take place during extreme weather conditions, will you be more comfortable with a portable heater, air conditioner, of fan in the room?

10. Do you have the name and phone number of at least one neighbor whom you would feel comfortable calling in an emergency?

11. Do you have important names and phone numbers of your doctor(s), hospital, relatives, friends, and work numbers for your partner next to the telephone?

Important Phone Numbers To Have Available:

_____

_____

_____

_____

_____

_____

_____

_____

_____

_____

_____

_____

_____

_____

Items To Make Your Bedrest More Comfortable And Convenient

There are several other items that you may find helpful in planning your bedrest space. Some of these things you may already have. If not, check with family and friends about borrowing them. Some items may be worth purchasing.

Bed tray – especially if you are able to eat in a semi-sitting position. Consider two trays so that a family member or friend can eat meals with you.

During my second pregnancy, Kelly bought me a folding wooden bed tray. It was sturdy and cost less than $15 – perfect for my meals in bed.

Cordless telephone – If you don't own one, this may be an excellent excuse for you to purchase a portable phone. It would be wise for you to carry the phone with you...even on short trips to the bathroom. An answering machine or automatic answering system is also a great help.

On one particular occasion I was in the bathroom when the phone rang. Five minutes later, the phone rang again and I was still sitting (pregnancy-induced constipation). Neither caller left a message on the answering machine. Five minutes later the phone rang again and I was able to answer. It was Kelly and he was frantic with worry that something was wrong. I learned that I needed to take the phone with me. This also came in handy when I was expecting my doctor's office to call.

A large nightstand or table – I have heard of women who bring the ironing board in and place it alongside their bed. It offers a lot of usable space and can be easily adjusted to be at the correct height.

A legal-sized clipboard with a hook on the top of it that could hang near your bed, or a notebook. This will be valuable for record keeping.

I monitored fetal activity four times daily, charted contractions whenever I felt that I was having more contractions than my hourly limit, and kept record of my medication doses. After I was on the Terbutaline sub-cutaneous pump, I also kept all of my records of syringe and site changes and daily infusion totals on my clipboard. It was helpful to have all of this information accessible for telephone calls with my doctor, nurse, or home-care nursing staff. I learned that tying a pen through the hole at the top of the clipboard was helpful.

Intercoms, walkie-talkies, or a baby monitor are all good ways to maintain contact with others in the house. If you are on one level of the house and your family is on the other, you will all appreciate having a means of communication. If you need help, you need only talk into the speaker to be heard.

Additional bedding – If you choose to create your bedrest space in the bedroom, as most women do, consider an egg-crate mattress. Many department and discount stores sell a variety of mattress pads. If your doctor orders a therapeutic mattress pad, your insurance carrier may cover it. If you are hospitalized for even a short period of time, you may be given an egg-crate mattress to bring home. You will also find extra pillows helpful. If you are not required to lay completely flat, you may wish to have a couple of pillows under your head and shoulders when you eat, and you will also want pillows behind your back to support you as you lay on your side. As your pregnancy progresses, a pillow strategically placed under your belly provides support.

My mom bought me a four foot long Body Pillow that I placed behind me during the day. At night, since I had to sleep on my left side, I used the pillow to wedge between my knees and under my belly.

High quality sheets – If you don't already own some, now is the time to indulge yourself with high quality sheets. Many people sleep on stiff sheets that contain a high percentage of polyester. One hundred percent cotton is a true luxury, although they will need to be washed three or four times before you want to sleep on them. Jersey-knit or flannel sheets are also very comfortable.

A shower chair – Assuming your doctor permits you to shower, you may wish to consider renting or purchasing a shower chair – a waterproof stool that sits in the tub allowing you the pleasures of a warm shower without having to worry about slipping. A rubber bath mat with a strong suctioned back is also effective. If you choose this option, you can purchase a hand-held shower attachment.

Meal Preparations And Food Concerns

Snacks And Meals For Bedresters

If your doctor allows you to prepare your own meals, you will need to plan for quick, easy, and healthy items. Obviously, this is largely a matter of personal taste, but it will still take some planning and organizing. Since you are probably not allowed to grocery shop, menu planning and comprehensive grocery lists for your partner are essential. There are many foods that are quick, easy, and healthy for you and your developing baby. Always plan for two snacks each day, and try to make them healthy, such as cheese and crackers, fruit, veggie sticks, granola bars, and breads. My weekly grocery lists always included the following food items for breakfast, lunch, and snacks.

- Yogurt
- Fresh fruits/vegetables
- Cheeses and crackers
- Peanut butter
- Whole-grain breads/bagels
- Milk
- Juices (preferably without added sugar)
- Granola bars

If your doctor will not allow a brief trip to the kitchen, your partner will need to stock a cooler or dorm-sized refrigerator for you. Even if you are allowed a couple of brief trips to the kitchen, save these trips for your meals by keeping snacks and beverages in your cooler and on your bed table. This is a great time to make use of commuter style mugs with sipper lids and large thermal water bottles with built-in straws. Drinking beverages in bed is not easy!

I had Kelly buy a six-pack of bottled water and after the bottles were emptied, he filled them with drinking water and stocked them in my refrigerator. I tried to drink all six bottles of water each day, since that was recommended. If you are using a uterine monitor you most likely already know how often the medical staff recommend the cure-all, "Drink a large glass of water, urinate, monitor for an hour, and then call me back."

Helping Your Partner With Meal Preparations

Kelly usually returned home from work by 5:30, so he prepared the dinner meal for us to enjoy together. It was helpful to have a weekly menu. It made grocery shopping and grocery list preparation much easier. It was also easy for him to look ahead to the following evening's meal and take any necessary ingredients out of the freezer for thawing. I became interested in healthy, well-balanced dinners that could be prepared in 45 minutes or less. I had some ideas in my recipe file and I also had Kelly choose some helpful cookbooks at the library. I spent countless hours looking for new, easy, nutritious recipes to try. (I also found plenty of fun recipes to copy and save for my triumphant return to the kitchen.)

A Crock-Pot can be a wonderful help to bedresting moms because it cooks food slowly over a period of 6-10 hours. In the morning, simply place some meat and vegetables in the Crock-Pot along with some type of liquid, such as stewed tomatoes, or a can of condensed soup. By dinnertime, your meal will be ready. A Crock-Pot produces flavorful, tender meats and delicious soups.

Helping Your Partner With The Grocery Shopping

Because Kelly suddenly found himself doing the unfamiliar task of pushing a grocery cart, I learned the value of well-organized, detailed grocery lists. I discovered that planning menus and then detailing a grocery list actually saved us money over time. In fact, this is something that I still do today. I plan 10 dinners, and then organize my grocery list accordingly. For Kelly to be able to shop effectively (especially the first couple of times he shopped alone), I had to be specific about the items I wanted him to buy. This saved me a lot of frustration, and Kelly found it a much easier to shop.

If you are planning grocery lists for your partner, and your partner has not been involved in grocery shopping, these ideas will help you both. If you are particular about brands or flavors, specify that on the list. If you simply put yogurt on the list, you never know what you will get. You also need to consider the following details: the size of the package you want, the quantity, flavors, etc. This may seem unnecessary, but it will ensure getting exactly what you want.

Arrange the grocery list based on the layout of the market. If the list is in order, it's much easier to shop and mark things off. If you have a partner who is adept at grocery shopping, congratulations. My experience was a lot different.

Kelly often came home with incorrect items, missed items, and flavors and varieties that suited his taste, rather than mine. I responded less than gracefully. It was difficult for me to let go of the responsibility, and my whining and complaining was unfair to Kelly. After a couple of stressful returns from the market, Kelly never questioned why my grocery lists were so detailed. (He quickly learned to buy only ice cream that had at least one type of chocolate in the title!)

Time-Saving Tips

Once you and your partner develop a meal and menu system that works for you, you may want to consider preparing double batches of casseroles, stews, soups, spaghetti sauce, chili, pre-formed hamburgers and turkey burgers, and even homemade muffins and cookies. Eat half of what you prepare and freeze the other half. You will be grateful for those frozen meals at other times.

And, never underestimate the value of leftovers. If you are limited to the amount of time you are allowed to spend on your feet, you will be grateful to have a plate of last night's dinner waiting for you to simply reheat in the microwave. Consider purchasing a microwave plate with three sections so your partner can prepare your lunch for you when the leftovers are put away. This is more cost effective, nutritious and better tasting than commercial frozen dinners.

After you and your partner have determined what your budget will be (especially if you are suddenly living with a reduced income due to your pregnancy bedrest), you will know better how much money there is for take-out and order-in meals. It will be a nice break for you to know that you will have pizza, Chinese take-out, or deli sandwiches occasionally. If you have friends and family members who offer to come and visit during the day, you might suggest that they stop for burgers or take-out on their way so you could enjoy lunch together. Eating alone can get old, especially if you are accustomed to eating lunch with a group of work associates.

What to Do With Your Time

Organizing Your Time While On Modified Bedrest

If you are on modified bedrest, your time resting can never be compromised. In fact, you have to allow for days when you are not feeling your best and will need to stay in bed all day. After you have a clear idea of the activities and household chores that you are able to participate in, your biggest challenge will be to determine your priorities for each day. For example, if you are allowed 10 minutes of activity per hour, try to plan what you can realistically accomplish in that 10-minute period of time so you are never pushing yourself.

During my second pregnancy, I spent two months on modified bedrest, adhering to the 10/50 rule (10 minutes of light activity and 50 minutes of resting). What helped me the most was a system of organization. Because I was able to accomplish small tasks, I felt less frustrated when it was time to go back to bed. Otherwise, 10 minutes just doesn't allow the opportunity to complete much.

For example, if you are allowed to perform light housecleaning, divide your tasks into small segments that are each approximately 10 minutes long. Maybe start by dusting. Instead of dusting your entire house, you will need to dust one room, or one section of one room, each time you have 10 minutes of activity. This system also works quite well for laundry. Assuming, of course, that you have verified with your doctor that you can bend and lift small batches of clothes. (You should always ask your partner to carry the baskets of laundry to and from the laundry room.) It shouldn't take more than 10 minutes to start a load of laundry. By the time your next activity break occurs, it will be time to transfer the laundry to the dryer and start the next load. By the following hour, one load will ready for folding. (Sit on a chair next to the dryer, and place the folded clothing into the laundry basket – don't carry it.) The other load will be ready for the dryer. If you plan your time, you will be surprised at how much you can accomplish. If you are on modified bedrest, you still have quite a lot of time to fill, and you may want to consider some of the ideas in the following section.

If you are on complete bedrest, the remainder of this chapter is written for you. Many of the following ideas may sound ridiculous. But when you are confined to bed for many weeks, you become easily excited about anything that will consume your time, and possibly even stimulate your brain.

Activities

Crafts

If you are an avid crafter, this is your time to work on all of those projects that you haven't had time to finish. If you have never been interested in craft projects, or if you simply haven't had time to explore the possibilities, now is the time. As I have already mentioned, it is essential that you be clear about what types of activity your doctor will permit – even in bed. If, for example, you are confined to lying on your left side, you will have to determine what you can realistically do.

When I was initially put on bedrest with my first pregnancy, I decided to teach myself counted cross-stitch. I spent several hours each day working on projects. I made gifts that were special to people because they understood that I had worked from my bed to make them. In the beginning, I asked my doctor for permission to go to the craft store. I spent about 30 minutes selecting books and the corresponding flosses and canvases. As my pregnancy progressed, Kelly was my craft store liaison. I would write down the numbers of each floss I needed, and he would go and pick them up for me. He was supportive of my activities and knew that I needed to keep myself busy.

If you know of a specific activity that you would like to begin, ask your partner or a friend to go to the store and select several different books for you. If you keep the receipt, most stores will allow you to return the items you don't want. (Ask about their return policy and have the shopper explain your situation.) Most craft stores are also willing to help you over the phone. When I needed a specific type and size of canvas, I called the store, asked them to prepare it for me, and Kelly just stopped in and picked it up. You will be amazed at the help you can receive by simply asking. Here are some craft ideas:

- Counted cross-stitch
- Stamped cross-stitch
- Latch-hook rugs
- Embroidery – there are many small, beginner kits available for simple projects like bookmarks or small wall hangings. Once you have learned the basic types of stitches, you are ready to venture on.
- Fabric painting on clothes, bibs, aprons, etc.
- Origami – (Origami is a beautiful method of Chinese paper folding. Your local library would have an instruction manual to help you get started.)
- Bead crafts – beading is easy to learn. Try a simple project like earrings or a barrette to start.
- Stamping with rubber stamps (consider stamping your own cards or stationery.)
- Crocheting or knitting – there are step-by-step instructional booklets available, many with photos that will help you start.
- Calligraphy – there are books to self-teach the different styles and strokes.

Television And Videos

Yes, it's true; television is a source of entertainment. There were many days when I had the television on while I was working on something else. I liked hearing the voices because it kept me from feeling alone. We also installed cable as soon as my first bedrest started. I was happy to be receiving so many movie and informational channels. Kelly moved our VCR into the bedroom and I would look ahead to see if there were going to be any old movies on after midnight – there always were – and I'd set the VCR and have a movie to watch the following day. Many cable companies offer packages for new subscribers and other special offers.

If cable is not an option, consider a membership at your local video store. There are several that offer memberships that pay for themselves quickly, especially if you rent videos several times per month. A membership may also entitle you to choose several movies, and then keep them for three or four days. A membership usually allows you the opportunity to call and reserve a copy of the new popular releases. As a change of pace, consider renting or purchasing videos about pregnancy, childbirth, infant care, or relaxation.

Reading

Bedrest will offer you the opportunity to read all of those books that you have never had time to read. The library may be a safe, simple excursion, if your doctor permits it. If you are totally confined, ask your doctor if you can go to the library for 30 minutes every couple of weeks. I was unable to, but my husband would bring home lots of books and I would simply choose the ones I was interested in. Many libraries now offer an on-line service – meaning that a complete library listing is as close as a home computer. You can also use your home computer to reserve books. Libraries may either call you to inform you that your selection has arrived or send you notification in the mail. If this is your first baby, it might be fun to check out some of the many books on baby care, child development, and psychology. There are also audiocassette books, movies and informational videos available for you to borrow.

Magazines are another good source of reading material. You could start a new subscription, particularly if you already know that your bedrest will be lengthy. Ask your friends and family members to save their magazines. I was always grateful for any magazines, even if they were several months old.

If you do not subscribe to the daily newspaper in your town, this is another idea for providing yourself with a consistent supply of new reading material. Several national newspapers may also be available for delivery. If you have never taken the time to attempt the puzzle page of the newspaper, now is a good time to start.

If you enjoy puzzle books, this is a great way to pass the time. Ask your partner to pick out some challenging crossword or other puzzle books of interest to you. There are many puzzle book companies that offer subscriptions. I inquired about a particular book and was granted a six-month subscription. It was a great way to keep my mind stimulated, further my vocabulary, and challenge myself to complete each puzzle book before the next one arrived.

Socializing

Once your friends and family members become aware of your situation, many will ask to come and visit. There may be people who are nervous about coming to see you because they do not understand your situation, or they are concerned that they could somehow further complicate your pregnancy. You and your partner need to decide whom you wish to tell, and what you want to tell them.

If you are early in your pregnancy and fearful you might lose your baby, maybe you won't wish to talk about your situation or have visitors. Or, you may find great comfort in having others around. You and your guests need to be aware that while you may welcome visitors into your home, you cannot assume the role of hostess. This is difficult because it is only natural to be concerned about the condition of your home and your ability to serve beverages and food to visitors.

Invite people at your own discretion. You are on bedrest because there is a complication with your pregnancy that could be dangerous for you and your baby. People may not realize what your limitations are. Women who have had healthy pregnancies are often surprised at the limitations. You need to feel comfortable explaining to people that you would love to have visitors, but that you will need to stay in bed.

Invite your guests to help themselves to snacks or beverages, but stay in bed. Don't hesitate to ask a guest to leave if you are feeling poorly. Most people truly want what is best for you and your baby, but they may need to be told exactly what that means for you. Your friends may assume that since you are in bed all day, you want guests to stay for a long period to help you pass the time.

I quickly discovered that even socializing and visiting was exhausting for me, and I was not always comfortable enough to ask guests to leave after I had tired. This only made my life more difficult because I was sure to have a rough evening if I didn't rest enough during the day.

It may be helpful for you to arrange a calendar if you have lots of friends and family members who wish to come visit. You may decide you don't want to have more than one visitor in a day, or no guests on the days you will be going to the doctor. It may be helpful to plan for guests only when your partner is home.

Kelly and I tried to invite friends or family to our home during the weekend since we enjoyed socializing as a couple. We would often order pizza. A few times our friends and family came with dinner for us. We would watch a movie or play cards while I lay on the couch. Those evenings did wonders for my spirits and I found myself looking forward to weekends for this reason.

I grew comfortable sharing my situation with people. During my first pregnancy, while I was on the Terbutaline sub-cutaneous pump, I was also using a home uterine monitor twice daily. I had to monitor at 9:00 each evening and then send the data to the home nursing company. My guests realized that my pregnancy took priority and were not at all surprised when I needed to change a terbutaline syringe or use my monitor. In fact, most were interested and amazed at the medical technology available to me.

Preparing For The Baby

If this is your first baby, you may feel frustrated at your inability to get out and buy furniture, clothing, and other supplies for your baby. It was a tremendous loss for me that I was unable to shop for our baby.

Kelly shopped for most of the clothing items we needed. One day he came home from the store so proud of himself because he had bought baby clothes for the first time in his life. He had selected all of the newborn layette clothing. As he pulled things out of the bags to show me, I started sobbing. This was my baby and I wanted to be the one selecting little onesies and T-shirts. Kelly felt so badly, and then I felt terrible for taking away his sense of joy and accomplishment. It was one of the many aspects of bedrest that I was forced to accept and deal with.

There are some things that you can do to prepare for the baby. In Chapter 11 you will find a list of businesses that have internet web stores or that will send catalogs so you can shop for your baby through the mail. Though you may still wish you could select items in person, it will give you the opportunity to shop yourself while occupying some of the time that passes so slowly in bed.

If you are thinking about sending birth announcements after the baby's arrival, now is the time to start thinking about them. If you are going to design the announcements yourself, start now.

Kelly and I designed our own birth announcements for both of our boys. I started a rough design during each of my pregnancies. We knew, both times, that we were having boys. Kelly went to the printer, selected the stationery, and purchased the envelopes. I spent two days addressing envelopes, putting on the return address stickers, and stamping them. This saved a lot of time after the baby was born since all that was left to do was write in the date of birth, time, and measurements. Kelly then dropped the announcement off at the printer and it was ready two days later. If you are going to purchase birth announcements, you can do that now as well. If you do not know the sex of your baby, there are plenty of birth announcements that are appropriate for boys or girls. I enjoyed this project because it helped me focus on the birth of a healthy baby.

It is also a great time to purchase or design baby thank you cards. You will have lots of notes to write after your baby arrives and after you have a baby shower. It may sound presumptuous, but I pre-addressed thank you notes to our family members and closest friends. This, too, saved me time after the baby was born. All I had to do was write the notes.

Other Projects

Paying Bills

If you have always handled your family finances, your bedrest will give you more time for paying bills and balancing accounts. If your partner has been the primary financial manager, you may want to consider taking over this responsibility since your partner will be busy with other responsibilities. If you have a reduction in income and/or additional expenses, you will probably be working with a budget. Your time in bed with the calculator will also give you the opportunity to start budgeting for the new expenses your baby will bring to your family: diapers, daycare (if applicable), clothing, feeding equipment and supplies, evening and weekend babysitting, as well as any furniture or other large purchases.

Volunteering

If you are active in your place of worship, consider offering your time for projects that you can work on from bed. You may be able to help with telephoning, or sending out correspondence. This is also useful for any other volunteer organizations you are involved in.

During my first pregnancy, Kelly and I were involved with a small nonprofit organization, and I participated in a couple of mailings. Kelly brought home the letters, envelopes, and stamps, and I did the work. Since the mailing was for a fund raising campaign, I also offered to write personalized thank you notes to contributors. I was happy to be contributing to the organization in a tangible way, and it really did save a lot of time for the coordinator.

Since I was also bedresting during a presidential election year, I called the League of Women Voters and offered to assist with a massive phone campaign to encourage people to get out and vote. I felt useful and believed that I was making a difference. It was a great feeling, since much of the time I felt like little more than an incubator.

Computers

There are many ways for you to access the world from a home computer. Technological advances offer some exciting ways for women on bedrest to educate, entertain, or communicate. Support and information can be found through web bulletin boards and chat rooms. There are many Internet sites for pregnant women, as well as various parenting web sites. If you are just starting out, I suggest using one of the search programs and entering key words such as "pregnancy." While there are many sites dedicated to parents, there are also excellent sites that will enable you to gain access to the most recent information pertaining to pregnancy and pregnancy complications. Chapter 11 includes a sampling of web sites.

Chapter Four

Surviving Bedrest In The Hospital

Pregnancy bedrest can be very stressful. If you are hospitalized for pregnancy complications, your frustration, anger, and sense of loss may be even greater. This chapter is intended to offer you some support and encouragement to cope with and survive these difficult days. I am writing this from my own experience with hospital bedrest. During my second pregnancy I was hospitalized for 11 weeks. Please be aware that every hospital is different, so some of my ideas and insights may not pertain to your particular situation.

I was at a large urban hospital that had an antepartal unit as part of the Birth Center. I was in the Birth Center, surrounded by the sounds (and screams) of women giving birth. I was also part of a camaraderie of pregnant women who were on bedrest due to severe complications in pregnancy, including PROM (premature rupture of membranes) pre-term labor, placenta previa, pre-eclampsia, and complications due to a multiple pregnancy.

If your doctor tells you that he wants to put you in the hospital, you will probably be shocked and frightened. The most important thing to remember is that your doctor wants you to deliver a healthy baby. You may be given a day or just hours to prepare yourself, your partner, and your family for this news. If you have children, you may need to find immediate care for them. You will need to notify your employer if you are employed outside of your home. Many women find that it is best to be as honest as possible in explaining the situation, so people are better able to support you and offer assistance.

Packing For The Hospital

You will want to pack items to take with you to the hospital. It is important to pack what you need to make yourself comfortable, both emotionally and physically. Some of the items to include:

- Nightgown and robe
- Slippers
- Socks, underpants, and bras (sport bras are comfortable when you are in bed all day)
- Your favorite pillow (in a bright pillowcase)
- Books or magazines
- A copy of the television viewing guide
- Your personal address/telephone book
- Stationery or note cards
- Any pregnancy books that you have (including this one!)
- Needlework, or other craft projects that can be done while you are in bed.
- Deck of cards
- Audio cassettes or compact discs with a small player
- Video tapes (call ahead to ask if you will have a VCR available in your room)
- Snacks, gum, or mints, as desired
- A small framed photo (or photos) of significance to you
- Ear plugs
- A small wallet or coin purse with change. It is wise to leave your checkbook and credit cards at home.
- A travel case or bag with your personal care items:

soap	shampoo
deodorant	hairbrush
hair dryer	toothbrush/toothpaste
cologne	dental floss
razor	cosmetics
lotion	lip balm
nail care items	hair accessories

_____

_____

_____

_____

_____

Settling In At The Hospital

Upon admittance to the hospital, you will have a wide range of questions regarding your care, particularly if you know that you will be hospitalized for more than a few days. Many of these questions should be answered for you by the nurse(s) who admit you and show you to your room. Some of these questions are more appropriate for long-term hospitalization, and are not necessary for women admitted for a short stay. Others cannot be answered until your nursing staff has more information about your situation. If any of your questions are not answered, feel free to ask the appropriate staff person. Immediately following this list I will look at each question individually and offer you some personal insights and ideas.

1. What are the visiting hours and are there any special provisions for my partner and/or children?

    _____

    _____

2. What are the hours at which my meals will be served and what is the procedure for ordering meals? What is the procedure for ordering or requesting snacks? Are there beverages and snacks available for my partner and/or children?

    _____

    _____

    _____

    _____

    _____

3. Does this unit validate parking for my partner? Is there a parking pass available for long-term hospitalizations?

    _____

    _____

    _____

4. What is the policy regarding additional support services, such as a social worker, psychologist, child psychologist, chaplain, etc.?

_____

_____

_____

_____

_____

_____

_____

_____

_____

5. What are the shift hours for the nurses?

_____

_____

_____

_____

_____

6. Based on my doctor's orders, what will be my daily routine?

_____

_____

_____

_____

_____

7. What is the policy regarding clothing? Am I required to wear a hospital gown at all times?

_____

_____

_____

_____

_____

8. What is the policy regarding my room? Can I bring pictures and wall hangings to personalize my room?

_____

_____

_____

_____

_____

_____

_____

_____

Visiting Hours

Some hospitals do not have specific visiting hours, particularly in the antepartal or obstetric units. But, if your hospital does, ask if they can be exempted for your partner (particularly if you are in a private room). Many women enjoy having their partner spend the night occasionally – a nice idea, particularly if you are hospitalized for a long period of time. The loss of physical closeness with your partner is a difficult aspect of hospitalization. If you have children, try to be mindful of the patients around you. It can be stressful hearing screaming children. Keep your door closed and remind your children that there are sick people who are sleeping and trying to get better. And be sure to tell your children that they must stay in your room.

On several occasions I had children wander in to my room and look around. The first few times this happened I was mildly amused. But as the weeks dragged on, and my stress levels rose, wandering children became a source of irritation.

Meals

Ah...hospital food. The hours at which your meals are served may not be negotiable. In most hospitals, you order your meals one full day in advance.

One of the highlights of my morning was deliberating over the menu for the following day. I will not waste a lot of space writing about how terrible some hospital food can be.

I will give you a few pointers which I learned the hard way.

1. If your food is not fit for human consumption, send it back. You are a patient who is eating for two and you deserve hot, relatively good tasting, food. Your nurses can help you return your food or they may give you the food service extension and you can call for a replacement item(s).

2. If an item(s) that you ordered is omitted from your tray, your nurses may have what you need. I learned that the nurses' lounge refrigerator was always stocked with milk, juice, and condiments. Another tip is to order double of certain condiment items and save them in your bed tray for a day when they are forgotten. Simply circle the food item and mark a "2" next to it.

3. Don't hesitate to request a copy of items which are routinely available from the hospital cafeteria, and make substitutions whenever necessary. I was given a list of cafeteria items, such as hamburgers, French fries, salads, deli-style sandwiches, and soups, which provided a nice alternative when the entree choices turn my stomach.

4. Ask a friend or family member to go to the cafeteria and write down some available food choices, and then request those items on your menu. For example, the hospital menu always offered three choices for dessert: fresh fruit, cookie of the day, and

something like tapioca pudding. However, the cafeteria offered fruit pies, fudge brownies and cheesecake. After a few weeks I finally decided that I had had enough bananas and tapioca pudding and started writing down "fruit pie" or "cheesecake" – surprise...I got it! This is also true for choices at the sandwich counter. Find out what types of meats and toppings are available and then request those items.

5. Ask your nurses which items in the cafeteria are good and which ones should be avoided. Granted, everyone has their own personal tastes, but you will be grateful to be forewarned about some of the really disgusting food choices.

I will never forget the hospital "Chicken A La King!"

6. If you would like a snack, your nurses should have a supply of milk, juices, soda, and various crackers and cookies available. You can also order snacks from the cafeteria and they will bring them at regular times. It's nice to have a small sandwich, or a muffin and fruit at bedtime.

7. There should also be coffee and soda available for your partner. Most nurses are happy to provide a beverage to make your partner more comfortable. As my weeks progressed, most of the nurses also got to know my son. When Will came for a visit, the nurses offered him juice and graham crackers – this became part of the ritual for him.

8. Ask your nurses if there are any local restaurants that deliver to the hospital. In the city where I was hospitalized, there were several options, including Chinese, Italian, and American. This will be a welcome departure. Order food and enjoy a (semi-) romantic evening with your partner. I heard of women who arranged for dinner to be brought in from nicer restaurants. They simply called the restaurant and explained to the manager their unique situation. One woman was able to arrange a surprise lobster dinner with her husband on the evening of their anniversary. Even pizza can be a wonderful treat – especially if you have a friend or family member to share it with.

9.   Don't hesitate to ask your friends or family to bring you something from a restaurant. If you are craving a Wendy's Frosty or a Big Mac, ask someone to bring it – most people will be happy to oblige.

One of my favorite nurses brought me a tomato and a cucumber from her garden and ordered me an extra large dinner salad. It was wonderful! My mom and my sister often brought me fruit or home-baked cookies and they always tasted better than ever before.

Parking

You should ask about parking validation for your partner. If you are hospitalized for more than a few days, ask if there are any parking permits or passes available.

Kelly was given a pass that enabled him to park for $1 per visit. The pass was issued for 30-day renewable intervals.

Support Services

While you are hospitalized, your doctor may order services from a physical therapist, occupational therapist, or a dietician.

There are many other services available to you that do not require a doctor's order. I received two or three visits from the child psychologist at the recommendation of one of my nurses. She offered me insights and advice about how to explain my situation to Will, and some ideas for Kelly to use when working with him at home.

There are always hospital chaplains available to provide counsel for patients. You can also contact your place of worship and request a hospital visit from your minister, priest, or rabbi.

Many hospitals offer support for women on bedrest, both at home and in the hospital. If your nurses don't mention any services for you, ask.

My hospital offered a program called "The Bedrest Connection," which was a group of trained volunteers (all with bedrest experience), who provided telephone support. Each new bedrester was paired with a volunteer who telephoned at least once a week to talk and offer support until the baby arrived. The hospital also offered a weekly support group that was run by a registered nurse with experience in obstetrics as well as her personal bedrest experience.

If your hospital does not offer support for bedresting moms, there may be other local hospitals that could refer you to support services in your area. There is also a national organization called Sidelines which offers support to women in high-risk pregnancies. Their phone number is listed in Chapter 11.

Nurses

As your days in the hospital progress, you will become more familiar with routines and schedules. Generally, nurses work an eight-hour shift, and then spend 30 minutes in "report" with the nurses coming on for the next shift. During report, each nurse reports the status of the patients that he/she has been responsible for, so that the new nursing staff is current about each patient's needs. If you buzz for a nurse during this time, it may take a bit of time for them to attend to you. Many nurses will come and ask you if you need anything before the end of the shift as a way of saying goodbye and letting you know that the shift is about to change.

If you are hospitalized for several days or weeks, your care will be handled differently by individual nurses. I learned that each nurse has their own gifts and talents that are reflected in how they conduct themselves. And, I discovered that it can take time to develop a relationship with a nurse. If you are hospitalized for a long period of time, you will most likely build wonderful relationships with your nurses and respect them for their unique talents and gifts.

Some nurses have a wonderful sense of humor and believe that laughter truly heals. Others have a gentle, caring spirit that enables them to reach out and offer support and encouragement. Some are professional and orderly, and will complete their responsibilities without a lot of personal involvement or conversation. You may also have nurses who seem insincere and not provide you with a level of care with which you feel comfortable.

I had many nurses that I came to love and admire. When it was finally time for me to move to Labor and Delivery, my departure was bittersweet. I was ecstatic about having the baby, but cried when I said goodbye to the staff. We had bonded and become part of each other's lives. We talked about marriage, child rearing, politics, religion, and shared personal aspects of our lives. It was difficult when that ended.

Finally, keep in mind that your nurses are there for you. Never hesitate to ask for anything that might make your stay, or your day, a bit better. Don't feel like you are bothering them. The best nurses will help you feel comfortable – asking what you need and helping you cope with your situation. If you experience problems with the nursing staff, discuss it with a nurse you can trust, or your doctor. They should be able to find out where to call and register a patient complaint.

Daily Routine

If you are going to spend more than one week in the hospital, daily routine will be important to you. Depending upon the specific complications in your pregnancy, you probably need to follow a schedule that the nurses help you determine. A daily routine is also helpful for a healthy state of mind, because you will feel like you have some control over your life. Include time for meals, personal grooming, and a shower/bath (if you are able), as well as time for monitoring or other daily tests that your doctor has ordered. You should also consider scheduling your visits from family whenever possible.

My days followed a pattern I was comfortable with. As the weeks progressed, my nurses all came to know my schedule, as well, so they were able to conduct their shifts based on the routines of their other patients. I depended on this structure and was grateful for the nurses who respected my desire to adhere to it. Whenever I was scheduled for an ultrasound or biophysical profile, I asked to be notified in advance so I could plan my day accordingly. I looked forward to my two or three biophysical profiles each week. I loved having an excuse to leave my room and go for a ride!

Clothing

Most bedresters are expected to wear hospital gowns. Because I was in the Birth Center of the hospital, I was given nursing gowns that came with two long slit-type openings on each side of the bodice. As my pregnancy and belly progressed, these gowns became quite revealing and the lovely floral design rapidly grew tiresome.

Because I was on an I.V., it would have been difficult for me to wear regular clothing. It was a time-consuming ordeal for my nurses to help me change my gown each day. But, I often wished that I could have worn some of my nice maternity clothes. I had several new summer outfits that were only worn a few times since I was hospitalized my entire third trimester. Wearing hospital gowns day after day became depressing.

If you are going to be in the hospital for several weeks you may wish to discuss the option of clothing with your nursing staff. Perhaps you could wear a nice outfit for one day each week, choosing a day when you are expecting company. Or, perhaps you could get dressed up to surprise your partner some evening, and ask if you could be taken for a wheelchair ride to the cafeteria for a soda or piece of pie.

You might lift your spirits by asking someone to buy you a new pair of comfortable slippers or a pretty robe. Some new hair accessories can also help you feel fresh. I know of women who brought their makeup to the hospital and felt better putting some on each day. Try to help yourself in the best way you can – find little ways to feel more human and make your days more tolerable.

Hospital Rooms

If you are spending several weeks in the hospital, ask if there are any guidelines regarding your room. Even if you are sharing a room, you still have a certain amount of wall space, a nightstand, or possibly a window ledge.

When I checked into the hospital, my nurses encouraged Kelly to bring pictures, or other momentos, to liven up my room. As the weeks progressed, I had a wonderful array of framed photographs from home on my window ledge. I also asked Kelly to bring a dried floral wreath which I had recently purchased. He hung it on a small nail directly across from my bed. Even my brightly colored pillowcases from home were a nice alternative to the heavily starched white hospital linens.

I heard of other hospital bedresters who brought a favorite blanket or quilt for their beds.

Keep in mind that you will be much more comfortable if you are able to surround yourself with some of your own belongings.

Other Ideas For Surviving Hospital Bedrest

In Chapter Three, I detailed some coping strategies for bedrest at home. Some of these strategies may also be helpful while you are hospitalized.

You may find that you are able to read or work on craft projects to help you pass the time. I met women who were crocheting, knitting, sewing, or cross-stitching quilts and blankets for their babies. I often thought what special meaning those gifts would hold as a reminder of their "days in waiting." Your partner, or a friend or family member, will be able to bring you all the necessary reading and craft supplies you need.

After you are more clear about your situation and how long you will be hospitalized, you can make some decisions about how you would like to spend your days. Your particular situation will dictate some of those things. Because I was on Magnesium Sulfate, I had a difficult time focusing my eyes, especially for the 48 hours after a level increase. As a result, I was unable to enjoy cross-stitching like I had during my first pregnancy. My Grandma shared copies of her large print books which made reading a lot easier. Libraries have a wide variety of large print books available as well as books on audiocassettes.

Since you will be watching a fair amount of television, ask someone to bring you a copy of the viewing guide from the Sunday newspaper. I often spent Sunday evenings looking ahead at the week's listings, circling the movies and specials I wanted to watch. It gave me something to look forward to during the week. If you have access to a VCR, movies are going to be a wonderful escape. There may even be a video library in your hospital. Video stores have various rental plans available and many offer you the option of keeping the videos for three or four days.

Kelly went to the video store on Tuesdays and rented five or six tapes for me which were not due until Saturday. Saturday night was movie night with Kelly and he often brought a special snack for us to share. My sister also came with videos and watched them with me. I also frequently looked at the cable listings and asked her to tape movies I was interested in seeing. I'm sure I watched at least 50 movies while I was in the hospital.

You will also need to make decisions regarding visitors. You and your partner need to decide whom you wish to inform of your hospitalization and how much information you want to disclose. Many women need to have their friends and family members involved during a difficult pregnancy. If you have other children, you will most likely require assistance from those people. But, there are some women who prefer to concentrate all of their efforts on their baby.

If you do not wish to have visitors, you need to discuss your feelings with your partner and decide how to best convey this to family and friends. While I was hospitalized, I was usually happy to receive visitors. I encouraged them to call ahead to make sure that I was having a good day and let me know what time they would be arriving. I was able to plan my morning and evening uterine monitoring, as well as my bath/shower time, around visits. I had days when I was not up to company, due to depression or frequent contractions, and I was honest with people and asked them to call another time.

Another problem you may encounter is visitors who stay too long. This was a difficult issue for me on more than one occasion. I knew that it was best to be honest, but I was so grateful for the company that I didn't know how to ask guests to leave. I tried subtle hints, but some people were not too perceptive. You need to realize that there will be visitors who have absolutely no idea what you are going through. People assumed that because I wasn't sick, and I was bored, that I would feel like having long visits. I actually had visits that lasted several hours and when the guests left, I felt exhausted. I talked with my nurses and developed a signal to let nurses know when I needed their assistance in asking my guests to leave. I would buzz the nurse's station and ask what time I needed to monitor. Since I never asked this question, (after all, I adhered to a schedule!) this let the nurses know I wanted my guest to leave. The nurse would then inform my visitor that it would probably be best for them to leave at this time. Although I felt badly for doing this, it really did help.

Another idea suggested by of one of my nurses was to close my door and put a sign on that said, "Mary Ann is sleeping. Please check with the nurses station." This gave me the privacy and time that I needed to be alone when I was having a really bad day.

I know the boredom, frustration, and depression that can accompany a hospital bedrest. But, I also know that each day of your hospitalization is a gift for your unborn child(ren.) This may be an excellent time for you to consider keeping a journal. Having a record of your days will be something you and your child will someday treasure. A journal can also help you process some of your depression and frustration. The days pass slowly and it can take a toll. I still have distinct memories of the depression, fear, and boredom that I lived with. My hospital gave all antepartal moms a pregnancy calendar to keep track of important milestones. I was not able to write very well because of the medications I was on, but I did chart the major milestones of each pregnancy. I am grateful to have one for each of my boys. You can create your own calendar or journal and record milestones as well as thoughts and concerns.

Above all, believe in yourself and your ability to cope with this situation. You can do this. You can survive hospital bedrest.

Chapter Five

Working With Your Doctor

T here have been many times in my life when I have looked into the faces of my two boys and felt tremendous gratitude for the miracles they are. As I reflect upon the journeys that led us to the birth of each of our sons, I realize that we would not be where we are today without the wisdom, guidance, and support of my OB/GYN.

The right doctor can make all the difference in your life, and ultimately, in the life of your unborn baby. I never doubted my doctor's decisions because I was so confident in his commitment to us. There were times when he was uncertain about the correct course of action to take, and we appreciated his honesty. We trusted his judgement, but no doctor can have all of the answers all of the time. When necessary, he obtained the advice and opinions of respected colleagues and specialists. A truly committed physician knows his/her limitations, and is not afraid to admit to a patient that he/she needs to seek the advice of someone more knowledgeable and experienced.

Every woman deserves a physician who will take the time to listen to her concerns, answer her questions, respect her feelings, and treat her with consideration and sensitivity. You will be working closely with your obstetrician (as well as other health care professionals) throughout your pregnancy to ensure the health of you and your unborn baby.

If you have been diagnosed as having a high-risk pregnancy, due to any of the various complications that can occur, your Family Physician, or OB/GYN may have already referred you to a specialist in high-risk pregnancies. If you are currently, or have recently been, hospitalized, you may have been examined by a staff Perinatologist. If your pregnancy complications are controllable by bedrest and/or medications, you may continue to be monitored by your regular physician. Regardless of who you are currently working with, it is important for you and your partner to feel completely comfortable with your doctor.

This may be the first time you need to be assertive with your physician. You deserve to have all of your questions and concerns answered. If you can't feel completely comfortable with, and confident in, your doctor, I would encourage you to consider finding another one. If you are not sure that you are working with the right doctor, there are some important questions to ask yourself. For example:

1. Does your doctor take time to listen to your concerns and answer all of your questions, without causing you to feel that he/she really doesn't have time for you? Does your physician try to minimize your concerns or feelings?

2. Does your doctor encourage you to call him/her, or the nurses, with any questions or concerns, regardless of the time of day or night? Are calls returned within a reasonable period of time?

3. Has your doctor said anything offensive to you regarding your pregnancy, your unborn baby, or the course of action you need to follow?

4. Do you feel that your doctor is doing absolutely everything that he/she could do to help you carry your baby to term?

5. Has your doctor reacted to your concerns and feelings with disinterest or insensitivity?

6. Does your doctor take time to talk with your partner and answer questions?

If you answered "no" to questions 3 and 5, and "yes" to questions 1, 2, 4, and 6, you probably have a strong relationship with a supportive doctor. But if these questions have given you cause for concern, you may wish to discuss with your partner what course of action is needed. It may be helpful for you to talk with your doctor about your concerns, or you may find the nurses at your doctor's office to be helpful in providing insights. They may be able to help you talk with your doctor about the type of care you are receiving.

Perhaps you would be wise to ask for a longer appointment slot for your next check-up. I know that many busy doctors have patients scheduled every 10 minutes. That is simply not enough time to answer questions. If you are scheduled for a longer appointment, your doctor may feel more relaxed and able to discuss your questions and concerns in greater detail.

If you have misgivings about your doctor, consider making an appointment with another doctor in the group. Each doctor in a group can have unique ideas and methods of treatment.

When I was pregnant with William, my doctor prescribed a Terbutaline subcutaneous pump. My doctor felt comfortable with this treatment, as it allowed me to leave the hospital and receive home-care from nurses. So, I was surprised to discover that two other doctors in the group were very opposed to the Terbutaline pump, and never prescribed it for their patients.

If you need the names of qualified physicians, contact the American College of Obstetrics and Gynecology (see Chapter 11) for a list of registered doctors in your area. They can also provide you with the names of OB/GYN's who specialize in Perinatology. Another source of information is friends and family. Most women are willing to share their experiences with their OB/GYN and can offer you a referral. Finally, you can contact one of the support agencies listed in Chapter 11 and request information about physicians.

Each doctor will have their own opinions and ideas about how to proceed with a high-risk pregnancy. If you are hospitalized for any length of time, you will most likely become accustomed to different doctors checking on you each day. While every OB/GYN group is different, it is common for each doctor in the group to be responsible for seeing hospitalized patients one day per week. You may encounter doctors who are outspoken about how they believe you should be treated, while others will prefer not to make any changes in your treatment plan. So, if you have any difficulties during evenings and weekends when your regular doctor is not on-call, remember that you will be speaking with another doctor, and need to take into account their unique personality and preferred treatment methods.

During my first pregnancy I was at home on bedrest and using the Terbutaline pump. On a few occasions, when I had difficulties and called the office, the on-call doctor seemed uncomfortable giving me advice since I was under the care of someone else. I was usually advised to go to the hospital. If this should happen to you, remember that your condition may not be serious, only that the on-call physician would feel more comfortable with you receiving care in the hospital until your own doctor is contacted.

Being An Assertive Patient

If you are hospitalized for a long period of time, you will need to be an assertive patient. In the beginning of a hospitalization there can be a lot of uncertainty. I found I needed to be especially assertive when another doctor attempted to make changes in my treatment plan that I was not comfortable with. Medicine is not a precise science and each problem can have several possible treatment options. Each doctor will have an opinion about which treatment is best for the patient. If you are being treated by a new doctor and about to receive an alteration in medication or procedure, it is both your right and your responsibility to be well-informed about:

- What is being prescribed?
- Why is it being prescribed?
- How could the drug or test affect you and your baby?
- Can it be avoided or delayed until you have had some time to consult your partner and your primary doctor?

As my hospitalization progressed, I was not responding to treatment, and my pre-term labor was not subsiding. My primary OB felt that he had done all that he could do for me and decided that it was time to consult a Perinatologist (a specialist who works with high-risk pregnancies.) The Perinatologist then formulated a treatment plan with my OB. I was informed of the options I had and was told what my doctors felt would be best. Once these options were explained, Kelly and I discussed them and realized that I would be wise to stay in the hospital on I.V. Magnesium Sulfate and receive Terbutaline shots when my contractions exceeded the acceptable number. As difficult as it was to accept, it was a blessing to know exactly what my treatment would be. I was no longer continually being given new options by different doctors. My OB and Perinatologist listed the specific orders in my chart so that every doctor who saw me knew what they were. On a couple occasions, a doctor would suggest something different, but this usually made me nervous. There was one doctor that I did not like, who frequently questioned the care I was receiving and the length of my hospitalization. He made inappropriate and hurtful comments that often brought me to tears. I finally expressed my concerns to my primary physician who asked that particular doctor to stop visiting me.

The nurses who cared for me also provided support as I worked with various physicians. Even knowing that my doctor took excellent care of me, that his schedule was full, and that I was only one patient, the hours passed slowly when waiting for him to come visit. On those occasions when I felt a stronger need to talk with my doctor, my nurse would call and ask him if he knew what time he would be coming. Just knowing he wouldn't be coming until later in the evening would allow me to relax a bit. I came to value the support of nurses who were willing to advocate for their patients.

Now is the time for you and your partner to assess your situation and decide whether you are satisfied with the care you are receiving. You deserve the best care possible. If you have any doubts, consider your options. In the days, weeks, and months to follow, you will need to feel completely confident in your doctor's decisions and be certain that everything that can be done for you and your unborn baby, is being done.

In conversations with other women, I found that high levels of confidence in their prenatal care was crucial for them. The greatest regret of one woman who delivered at 28 weeks was that she always felt her doctor was minimizing her complaints and not really listening to her concerns. She would always question whether the doctor could have done more to prevent her baby's two month hospitalization. She also shared she would find a new physician before becoming pregnant again.

I have also met many women who delivered early or endured difficult pregnancies who are truly convinced that every necessary precaution was taken. For these women, that level of confidence makes all the difference in their acceptance and outlook.

Chapter Six

Dealing With The Losses Associated With Bedrest

I n many ways, my bedrest pregnancies feel like another lifetime ago. But as I reflect on each bedrest they feel very recent, and the frustrations and hurt are surprisingly near. I wanted to write this chapter because I hope my honesty will be of some benefit to other women sharing this experience. It is a difficult part of my past, and I have had to take some time to deal with the losses I experienced, particularly while hospitalized.

Reading this chapter may or may not help you right now. Maybe you'll read it and have a sense of relief knowing you are not the only one experiencing these feelings. Or, maybe you will need to come back to this part of the book weeks, or months, after your baby has arrived and you are trying to move forward.

Whatever the case, I hope that my sharing gives you a sense of peace that you can survive this experience.

Loss Of Freedom And Control

Loss of freedom and control is the first reality of pregnancy bedrest and will most likely hit you hard during the first week you spend in bed. You no longer have the freedom to decide what you will do, how you will do it, where you will do it, and with whom you will do it. That sense of power and control is gone. If you are hospitalized, you cannot even decide when to eat, shower, or talk with your doctor. For many women, this is the first time in their

---

adult lives that they feel as if they have virtually no control over their lives.

All of us experience this, to a lesser degree, when we are ill. What usually helps us cope is the knowledge that the illness will last only a few days. Bedrest is usually not for just a few days. If you are facing several weeks or months on bedrest, the most valuable coping technique is simple: "Let go."

You will not be able to let go right away. You will feel anxious about every detail of your life and the lives of your family members. But that will only make your life, and possibly your pregnancy, more difficult. Each morning, remind yourself of why you are in bed, what your goal is, and how you are going to reach that goal. If you believe in the interventions of a higher power, now is the time to be seeking strength, patience, and endurance.

My faith sustained me through many long, sad days.

You will also discover that you will need to cling to the few bits of control you still do have. If you are home, taking responsibility for a few household tasks such as menu planning, bill paying, and grocery list preparation will enable you to feel in control over certain aspects of your life. Participating in these areas of household management will also alleviate some pressures put upon your spouse. It is ironic that while you are struggling with a loss of control and responsibility, your partner might be struggling with total control and responsibility. Communication will be the glue that holds you together. Discuss your feelings and listen when your partner shares with you.

If you are hospitalized, you are seemingly forced to give up control in every aspect of your life. The establishment of a daily schedule, as I discussed in Chapter 4, will restore some sense of control over your life. Ask your nurses and medical team to respect your desire for a consistent schedule.

It can be helpful to remind yourself that, ultimately, you *are* the one in control. I know that sounds peculiar, since you probably feel like your pregnancy is controlling you. But *you* are the only person who can decide to stay in bed and follow the doctor's orders.

Freedom is a much more difficult need to fulfill. If you are home on bedrest, your greatest freedom is from most responsibilities of career, family, and home. While this is not always a welcomed reality, it is still a freedom to try and enjoy, especially since after your baby arrives, it will be gone.

When I was home on bedrest with my first pregnancy, I stayed up until 2:00 a.m. watching old movies. I then slept until 11:00 in the morning, waking just in time to tune in to my favorite soap opera.

Never mind that you are required to spend your freedom in bed. As difficult as it may be, try to remind yourself of the luxuries your bedrest affords.

In the hospital I did not have many of the freedoms that I enjoyed at home. I began to consider some of the little things-like filling out my daily menu-as freedoms. I also enjoyed having nurses ask me when I would like to have my linens or I.V. site changed and what time I wanted to monitor. I had freedom and control in just a few small ways but, under the circumstances, they seemed significant.

Depending upon your situation, you may be allowed short wheelchair rides. Do not pass up this opportunity to get out of your room. After several days or weeks of looking at the same four walls, a short ride will seem liberating.

If you are like me, you may not have the luxury of wheelchair rides outside. After the first month of my hospitalization, my wheelchair rides were suspended due to the frequency, severity, and duration of my contractions. I will never forget walking outside on the day of my discharge. I had not breathed fresh air for eight weeks. I felt a sense of liberation and freedom that I had not experienced before- as though I had just walked out of prison.

The only way I could cope with my two bedrest pregnancies was to look for new opportunities to take control. The loss of freedom taught me to relax, enjoy life and let go of those things I could not control. To this day, I no longer take many of the every day freedoms for granted.

Loss Of Employment

If your bedrest requires you take a leave of absence from outside employment, this will most likely be frustrating. The first week may seem like a vacation, but as the weeks and months progress, you will find yourself feeling under-challenged and bored without the intellectual stimulation that your job provided.

During my first pregnancy, leaving my job also meant that I had to worry about the person who was assuming my responsibilities. I wanted to believe I was irreplaceable. Of course I wasn't, and that itself was an important lesson to learn. I also missed the personal interaction and friendships of my coworkers.

I was able to remain involved with work for the first few weeks of my bedrest. I worked on paperwork from my bed and my husband dropped off my work and picked up messages. I enjoyed remaining connected in that way. This may be an option for you to pursue, depending on your doctors' recommendations and the type of work you do.

While I was home on bedrest with my second pregnancy, I was forced to enroll two-year-old William in daycare. Although it had originally been a difficult transition for me to quit my job and be an at-home mom, I had been at home full-time since William's birth. But when I was forced to send him to daycare and spend my days in bed, I became miserably depressed. I realized my son absolutely loved going to daycare. While I knew I should be relieved, I felt the pangs of disappointment. Just like with my first pregnancy, I expected to be missed more than I was. Though I would have been far more upset if Will had not adjusted to daycare, it was difficult for me to admit that he didn't miss spending his days with me.

Bedrest may cause you to feel frustrated with your lack of productivity, and it's perfectly normal to feel you have become little more than a "human incubator." In reality, that is exactly what you need to be at this point. There is no job more important than that of nurturing your baby and you can take solace in knowing that nobody can do this job but you. In a few more weeks, or months, as you cuddle your beautiful newborn, you will fully realize the importance of this very special job. Keep up the great work.

Loss Of Social Life

Bedrest will force you to redefine your social life and how you, and your partner, define leisure time. This is particularly true if this is your first pregnancy. You may be accustomed to dining out, going to movies, concerts, theatre productions, sporting events, parties, or working out at the gym. You may have curtailed some of your activities at the beginning of your pregnancy, but bedrest will cause most, or all, of these activities to come to an immediate halt.

You and your partner will discover that a game of Monopoly or a rented video now seems to be the sum of your choices for how to spend a romantic, leisurely evening together.

It can be helpful for you both to invite friends over for an evening. Your friends will be more likely to understand, and offer their assistance, if you are open and honest about your situation. You must take care of yourself and stay within the guidelines that your doctor has ordered, so, if you are feeling tired, excuse yourself and go rest. Your partner needs to assume full responsibility for entertaining. You can make this easier by inviting guests to come after dinner, or by suggesting that you order dinner from a take-out restaurant. If your friends offer to bring dinner, accept. You need to learn to let people help.

Loss of your social life can be an added stress on your relationship with your partner. You need to discuss what types of activities your doctor will allow you to participate in, and make plans accordingly. You also need to decide what activities your partner can participate in without you. This is a difficult aspect of bedrest. You are forced to let go of so much in your life and need to occasionally let go of your partner, as well. Spending the evening in bed while he goes without you to a party or family event is, without question, a horrible experience.

I spent many nights crying and feeling sorry for myself. It took a lot of strength and love to tell Kelly that it was okay for him to go out without me. He was assuming so many new responsibilities and I knew he deserved some time for himself. During my second pregnancy, it was even worse for him. He had responsibility for our son while I was in the hospital. He wanted to spend all of his free time with me, but I had to be strong enough to encourage him to take care of himself, even if it meant that I wouldn't see him for the day. I recall one Saturday when my mom offered to take care of Will for the day. Kelly stayed home and was able to tend to household responsibilities and relax. He felt energized and refreshed after some time alone.

Loss Of Intimacy/Sexual Relationship

If you are on bedrest, your doctor should give you specific directions about what types of physical and sexual activities you are able to engage in. For many women, this means nothing. During both of my pregnancies, I had premature labor. Any type of physical stimulation, including kissing, increased my contractions. Kelly was forced to basically avoid touching me at all. Embraces were acceptable, but we were forced to keep them short. It was a difficult adjustment since, during our first pregnancy, we had only been married for six months when my bedrest started.

I know there are women on bedrest who are allowed some options for sexual expression. It may mean that you need to experiment together to determine what types of activities will permit you to remain within the boundaries that your doctor has ordered. You and your partner need to communicate openly during this time since it will most likely be a difficult adjustment for both of you.

Kelly and I were forced to redefine intimacy in our marriage. This turned out to be a positive thing for us. After being forced to remain celibate for several months, we started reaching out to each other in new ways. We developed an emotional, spiritual, and intellectual intimacy that became our lifeline. This not only gave us new meaning in our marriage, it also made the second pregnancy-induced celibacy easier to handle.

Writing love letters, watching an intellectually stimulating movie and then discussing it, or reading a book together and discussing it, can all be helpful ways of maintaining intimacy without sex.

Loss Of Parenting Time

If this is not your first baby you may be concerned about how your bedrest will affect your other child(ren.) My oldest son turned two when I was on bedrest the second time. I worried about how his needs could be met. Placing him in daycare was difficult, but I also knew it was the only answer. Will needed to be physically and emotionally fostered in ways that I was not able.

For you, the mother on bedrest, the most important thing is to accept the feelings that you are experiencing and then deal with them and move forward. I spent too much time feeling guilty. I tried to remind myself that Kelly and I were giving Will the gift of a baby brother, and we truly believed that we were doing everything possible for Will. But when I was hospitalized, I became depressed thinking about all the special moments I was missing over an entire summer with him. I still feel badly about that at times, but I also understand that I can't mourn the past.

For his part, William had a wonderful summer, and was able to spend time with his cousins, grandparents, aunts, and uncles. Many of these special times would not have happened if I had not been hospitalized. There were many blessings in our lives, and we were fortunate that William's summer was one of those positive experiences.

Whenever I started feeling depressed about my inability to mother my son, I concentrated all of my energy on mothering the son growing in my womb. There was a bittersweet irony in my life: I had to let go of mothering Will, so that I could mother and eventually give life to Colin. I worried about how Will and I would get along after the baby arrived, and reminded myself that each day was going to be a journey our family would travel together. I took solace and pride in knowing that Will had easily adjusted to all the changes in his life and that he was secure and happy in so many varied environments. I realized that I was raising a happy, well-adjusted child.

Loss Of Opportunity To Prepare For Baby

When I discovered that I was pregnant with my first child, it took great restraint to not rush out and buy a crib, stroller, clothing, and all the other necessities that a new baby requires. In the excitement, it seemed like nine months was such a long time to wait. Choosing nursery furniture, equipment and clothing is a special experience for expectant parents, particularly with their first baby.

If you are suddenly sent to bed, you may not ever have the opportunity to go out and shop for your baby. You may not be able to paint or wallpaper the nursery walls.

I was sent to bed in my 13th week of pregnancy with Will. The week before my bedrest began, Kelly and I had been out looking at houses and anxiously planning a move out of our apartment. Because my doctor ordered complete bedrest, we weren't able to move. We had to try to reorganize our den/home-office/computer-room to accommodate our baby. It was not at all what we would have chosen for our first baby.

My sister wanted to have a shower for me, but we knew we needed to wait until after the baby arrived. I was tremendously disappointed but realized my situation was not going to change, and I needed to accept it and make plans accordingly.

Kelly shopped for layette clothing, an experience he enjoyed. My mother made a baby quilt, and helped me coordinate crib linens. Kelly's brother and his wife gave us their changing table and baby swing. My sister also enjoyed shopping for baby items. And me? I stayed pregnant. I stayed in bed every day, and helped my baby grow stronger and healthier. I had the hardest job, was the only one who could do it, and I knew I had to do it well. That was the attitude I tried to maintain. I also knew that our new baby was not going to mind sharing space with a desk and a computer. A freshly decorated nursery was not the most important thing for our baby–a healthy start followed by lots of love and devotion from his parents was all that he would need.

There will be lots of time for decorating later on. (Chapter 11 is a list of shopping resources for all of you who need to shop from the confines of bed.)

Loss Of Income

Financial concerns may be a loss that is a painful reality, particularly if you and your partner depend on your income. If you know that your bedrest is going to be long-term, you may qualify for disability benefits. You should consult the personnel director at your place of employment and fill out the necessary forms. Many employers will allow you to use vacation or sick time compensation you have saved. I was able to apply the balance of my vacation time to the 30-day waiting period that was required to qualify for disability benefits. But disability benefits can vary greatly.

There is no question that you will need to evaluate your current budget and spending habits and determine where you can cut corners. If you are on total bedrest, your entertainment budget may be all but erased.

During my first bedrest, we were surprised to discover how much money we had been spending on movies and dining out. Our entertainment budget became a payment to the cable company, and an occasional pizza delivery. Our Christmas budget was slim that year, but our families were understanding. We decided to sell one of our vehicles and purchase a less expensive one. The difference in loan payments saved us $100 per month. We also dipped (deeply) into our savings.

During my second pregnancy, one of our greatest financial challenges was paying for William's daycare. We were fortunate to have the help of our families who knew that daycare was a financial burden and offered us a great deal of help. Kelly also began a job working sleep shifts at a group home. It meant that he was gone four nights a week, but the extra income was a necessity.

If your income is severely altered, and you are unable to cut enough of your expenses, you may need to consider borrowing money. If you have money available in the form of stocks, bonds, or an interest-bearing retirement account, you may be able to draw money from these sources. Or, you may want to consider a personal loan from a family member. Another option is talking with your banker. Perhaps a consolidation loan would enable you to combine your debts into a more manageable monthly payment. You may also qualify for an interest rate that is significantly less than the current rate on most major credit cards.

If you are acquiring new debt that is related to the pregnancy, talk with your healthcare provider(s) and ask if there are budget plans for persons who are having difficulty paying their bills. Our experience was that hospitals and doctors' offices are willing to set up a payment plan that is mutually agreeable.

Finally, despite the financial stresses, try to remain focused on the goal of delivering a healthy baby. You and your partner need to look at your monthly budget together to determine where your expenses can be cut and your income enhanced. If this is your first baby, you were probably already considering how your baby would affect your income and budget. Overcoming financial stress can strengthen your relationship while teaching you how to live on less – a very valuable lesson.

In Conclusion

Coping with the losses associated with pregnancy bedrest is difficult. It is important to realize that your partner and your children are also dealing with losses...especially the loss of your involvement in the day to day family activity. It is crucial that you and your partner communicate honestly about your natural and normal feelings of sadness, frustration, anger, and resentment. Whatever your feelings of loss, try to acknowledge and accept them, and determine how you can best manage them and move forward.

I found "journaling" to be a helpful way to process my feelings. I encouraged Kelly to talk with other people about how he was feeling. Sometimes we needed to talk with people other than each other, particularly when we were each feeling overly stressed.

Above all, remember that this experience is teaching you and giving you new insights. In the months and years that follow your bedrest experience, you will often recall the struggles you endured and feel proud of your ability to accept and cope with the challenges you were given.

Chapter Seven

Helping Children And Families Understand Bedrest

I f you have children, you have an additional challenge in caring for their needs while you take care of yourself. You may be wondering how you will handle the difficulties in balancing their physical and emotional needs with your own.

Many women are blessed with friends and family who offer assistance during a difficult pregnancy. But the support that bedresting women receive varies considerably. I have met women who found the lack of support from family and friends to be a source of disappointment, anger, and deep hurt.

This chapter is intended to offer ideas for helping your children through this challenging time, and to offer some words of wisdom for those of you who are disappointed with the response you are receiving from people you thought you could count on.

Helping Your Children Understand Bedrest

Your doctor should have given you specific limitations and guidelines with regard to your children and the level of care you are able to provide. Please take that into consideration when you are reading this chapter.

My son, Will, was a month away from his second birthday when I began my second bedrest. My husband and I weren't prepared for the ways we would have to help Will adjust to the changes in his life.

My bedrest was modified for about 6 weeks, so I was able to care for Will for part of the day, and I hired a couple of college students to care for him for 2-3 hours daily. They were wonderful about taking him outside and running with him to vent some of his energy. The rare days that he napped were also a blessing. Kelly also tried to work shorter days, bringing work home to finish after Will was in bed.

During my time with Will, I positioned myself on the couch and tried to keep him entertained while lying down. We developed new ways of playing with his toys and he enjoyed being my special courier who brought me toys and books. We soon developed a schedule which seemed to benefit both of us.

If you are trying to care for your children while on modified bedrest, I highly recommend a schedule. A routine will help your children accept the breaks you need to take, especially if they know the schedule includes other times for play.

Getting out of the house seemed to make the days pass more quickly for both of us. Will and I enjoyed lunch at fast-food restaurants and rides in the van. Because of his young age, he was easy to entertain, but his attention span was brief.

I will always remember our trips to watch construction workers as they built a new video store. Will was fascinated by the construction vehicles and we could sit for an hour and just watch and discuss the different trucks and what they were used for.

Here are some other ideas for passing the time with your children while you are on modified bedrest. Bear in mind your doctor's orders and limitations. If (or when) your doctor orders complete bedrest, many of these activities will no longer be possible or practical.

Entertaining Your Children While On Modified Bedrest

- Playing outside before a nap helps to get the wiggles out.
- Board games/flash cards/card games are always fun – an ironing board works well as an adjustable bedside table.
- Consider cable television, and subscribe to children's programming stations.
- Let your child play doctor with a juvenile doctor's kit.

- Play-dough/modeling clay.
- Build with Legos/Duplos.
- Work on puzzles
- Pretend your bed is a tent, and tell stories under the covers, using flashlights.
- Have fun with coloring books, crayons, and colored pencils.
- Offer to give a manicure.
- Rent videos, borrow them from the library or from your friends and neighbors'.
- Read books or listen to books on tape.
- Make audiocassettes with your children singing, telling jokes, or reading books.
- Practice skills such as printing, handwriting, saying the alphabet, addition/subtraction, etc.
- Play "20 Questions" or "I Spy".
- Telephone a friend or grandparent each day.
- Consider teaching a new craft such as crocheting, embroidery, or fabric painting.
- Ask your doctor how often you can sit or lay outside so your children can still get some exercise.
- By all means...rest when your children are resting.

And...if you can drive:

- Go to a fast-food restaurant for lunch, a soda, or an ice-cream cone. The places that have an indoor playground are great.
- Visit friends or relatives.
- Go to the movies.
- Go to the library – try and time your visit with "Storytime".
- Go for a ride...anywhere.

It will be important for you and your partner to try to help your children understand your limitations. For most bedresting women, the evening is the most important time to rest in bed because it is often easier to do when your partner is home.

For Kelly and I, the evenings were a great time for me to go to bed and rest. Unfortunately, Will didn't understand why I was continually resting at night, and he often complained and cried at bedtime because Kelly was the one always putting him to bed. We soon revised our routine, and Will came to my room for stories after he was ready for bed. This was a nice way for us to end our day.

Mothering While On Complete Bedrest

I know of women on complete bedrest who do try to care for their children at home. This is a decision that you and your partner will need to make with your doctor's input. Most often, however, complete bedrest usually precludes caring for your children. I know that being told you cannot care for your children is a difficult thing to hear, and even more difficult to accept and adhere to.

For me, after six weeks of modified bedrest, my doctor said he did not want me caring for my child by myself, and I was put on complete bedrest. I was devastated. After exploring daycare options, we enrolled Will in a full-time Montessori program. I was still upset that I was not the one offering William the care he needed, but I realized the school offered him many beneficial opportunities. And, most importantly, I was able to relax and concentrate on my pregnancy knowing that Will was in good hands. He was happy to go to school and sometimes even disappointed when it was time to return home.

After my situation worsened, we knew that moving closer to our families was the best option for everyone. When it became apparent that I would be spending the summer in the hospital, I was grateful for the support and assistance that our families offered us in caring for Will. Being separated from him for 11 weeks was difficult emotionally. There were many days and nights when I could only cry. I missed the bedtimes, the meals, the snuggles, and the adventures of life with my two year-old.

However, he had wonderful times with his dad, cousins, aunts, uncles, and grandparents. Will's relationship with his dad blossomed while I was hospitalized, and that was a blessing for them both. A stronger relationship between fathers and their children seems to often occur while a mom is on bedrest. But it can be difficult to realize that your children do not have the same relationship with you that they once had. After Colin was born and we all moved back home, it took some time for William and I to find our mother/child relationship again...but it happened.

I know that I missed an entire summer with Will, and that is time lost forever. Sometimes when I watch my children play in the warm sunshine or splash in their pool, I remember the summer of hospital bedrest and feel sadness about the time I lost with William. But then I look at Colin and know that he is here because of that summer in the hospital.

I know now that I spent too much time worrying about William while I was hospitalized. My pregnancy hormones were in overdrive. I had nothing else to do with my time, and the medication affected me. As I reflect on that time, I realize just how resilient Will really was. He adapted well to the changes and seemed to accept the situation. When he was leaving the hospital at night he often asked if I could come home. That was difficult for Kelly and I, but we always tried to explain that I had to stay in the hospital so the baby could grow bigger. And, we always reminded him that I would be coming home after the baby was born. He seemed most concerned that the intravenous bags and tubes might be hurting me. We explained that the bags were filled with mommy's special medicine to help the baby stay inside my tummy and grow. Other than that, William seemingly enjoyed the adventures of his unpredictable life.

I know that others with older children had a more difficult time answering some of the questions their kids asked them, especially while hospitalized. Most tried to help their children understand that there were problems with the pregnancy and that bedrest was the best way to keep the baby safe. It seems easiest to focus discussions on the baby since that is something the children are already anticipating. Telling a child that "the baby wants to come out too soon" and that "bedrest helps the baby grow bigger," are common explanations. Children of all ages benefit from honesty and it is up to you and your partner to decide what is the best explanation to offer. It is important that your children feel comfortable asking you questions or discussing their feelings. Older children may have concerns and worries about the health and safety of the baby, or of you (especially if you are hospitalized) since children tend to equate hospitals with sickness. Many children need constant reassurance that you will be coming home after the baby is born or that your bedrest will end after the birth. If you think that an early delivery is possible and that your baby may spend time in the neonatal intensive care unit, you will need to decide how and when to discuss that with your children.

Hospital Visits From Your Children

If you are hospitalized, you and your partner will need to make decisions about visits from your children. If you are expecting to be hospitalized for more than a week or two, you may wish to devise a schedule, since that will benefit everyone.

The hardest thing to accept is that it may not be realistic for you to have a visit from your children every day. School activities, work requirements, and the distance you live from the hospital will all be factors that determine visits. Sometimes it takes a lot of trial and error to determine the best schedule. Younger children can't be kept entertained for long periods of time, and unfortunately, their visits may be stressful for you, particularly if they are upset. A visit from your children can remind you that you are needed and missed. Seeing them frustrated, sad, or angry can cause feelings of anger, guilt, and depression.

An hour or less is usually the longest visit a young child can handle, while older children might stay longer. For all children, however, it is best to plan for the visits. Make certain that you understand your limitations and then consider some of these ideas:

- Color together on your bed tray (make sure you have a good supply of coloring books and crayons)
- Have a bucket of Duplos handy.
- Read stories (consider purchasing a couple new books to keep at the hospital).
- Coordinate visits with a favorite TV program.
- Watch a special video together...(maybe buy a new video to keep at the hospital).
- Have a snack together. (Ask your nurses for crackers, cookies, and juice).
- Order a pizza for dinner some evening. (Order it ahead of time, to minimize the wait).
- Inquire about a playroom with toys you may be able to visit (common in hospitals with a children's wing).
- Have your partner take your children to the nursery-viewing window to see the new babies. It may help prepare younger children for the new baby, while reminding them of why mommy is hospitalized.

- Plan bathtime in your room, even if you can only watch while your partner gives a bath. Help your children get their pajamas on and read stories before they leave.
- Invite older children to come when you are having an ultrasound.
- Play a board game (suitable for older children).
- If you can arrange a wheelchair ride, plan a walk outside or a trip to the cafeteria.
- Encourage school-aged children to bring their homework assignments and papers to share with you.
- If you have a foldout bed in your room, older children may be able to spend a night with you.
- Consider keeping special books or toys in your room so children will have something familiar when they visit.

It is also a good idea to schedule some individual visits if you have more than one child. Recognize their differing needs. An older child may need time to just talk with you, while a younger child will be more interested in engaging in some familiar activities. Whatever you are doing, these times together will enable you to feel like you are still a mom to your children. Many moms I spoke with said that the time they spent reading, talking, and snuggling with their children were the happiest moments of their bedrest experience.

Finally, while hospitalized, you will soon discover the gift of the telephone in maintaining connections with your kids. Even if they are young, and not speaking clearly, you will be grateful to hear their voices and they will be thrilled to have received a phone call from you.

I faithfully called Will every day at 12:30 p.m. He talked constantly and I understood only about 25% of what he said, but it didn't matter. He thought I understood all of it and that's what mattered most to him. If he couldn't come to see me at night, he called me before he went to bed. Many routine bedtime struggles were eliminated because he was so anxious to call his mommy. Whenever he spent the night with someone else, he still called to say goodnight. This was important for both of us.

Helping Friends And Family Understand Bedrest

Pregnancy problems can develop quickly and if you suddenly find yourself on bedrest, you may wonder how to explain your condition to friends and family. Some people have never known anyone who had a problematic pregnancy, so the mere concept of bedrest is foreign to them. Others will be surprised and curious about your condition. As with any difficult situation, reactions will vary greatly.

It is not uncommon for people to seem uncomfortable hearing about your pregnancy problems. If you are in the first half of your pregnancy, people may be concerned about the risk of miscarriage, even though few will mention it. Some people, while trying to be helpful, will say something hurtful.

When I began bedrest with William at 13 weeks, I had placental abruption and was bleeding. We knew I was at high risk for miscarriage. One of my relatives' response was, "You're young...if you lose this baby, there will be others." I cried most of the afternoon. A couple of people asked me if I had "done something to make this happen?" Again, I cried. Another horrible comment was "maybe this baby just isn't meant to be."

It was difficult to try and explain our situation to others. The first pregnancy was the hardest because for three months we were filled with fear that I would miscarry. Most of our friends and family offered emotional support. During the first weeks of bedrest I had a lot of company - my visitors felt badly and wanted to show their support. Then the visits started to lessen, the phone calls were fewer, and I wondered if people were starting to forget about me. It seemed the only days the phone rang were those that I had a doctor's appointment because a few family members were good about calling to check on my progress.

There were friends and family who knew I was on bedrest and chose to do nothing. It was hurtful that they didn't call or send a note during 22 weeks of complete bedrest, but I assume they were just too uncomfortable with our situation to deal with it.

I often heard comments like, "I'd love to spend my days in bed...it must be so relaxing to not have any responsibilities." Or, "I know that I could never deal with bedrest myself...I would just go crazy." I learned to try to see past the comments and look for the thoughts or feelings that a person may have been trying to convey.

Anyone who has ever experienced a death, serious illness, or other loss has experienced hurtful or unwelcome comments from well-meaning people trying to offer support. Kelly and I learned to accept and appreciate the ways that people reached out and we always tried to show our gratitude. As for the people who disappointed or hurt us? We tried to move past that too, and concentrate on the positive experiences.

When I spent a week in the hospital at the end of my second trimester, I was surprised at the amount of company I had. People seemed to go out of their way to visit, and I loved it. While Kelly was so happy when I was able to come home from the hospital, I soon became depressed because I no longer had visitors.

I didn't understand why people felt that it was more important to visit me in the hospital than at home. Perhaps they felt too uncomfortable inviting themselves to our house or they just assumed I wasn't as lonely at home.

So, Kelly and I started inviting people over. We invited friends to come on the weekends and we'd order a pizza and play cards or a board game. We explained my condition and treatment so our visitors could better understand why I needed to lie on the couch and monitor my contractions while we talked. If I was feeling uncomfortable, or my contractions were particularly strong, I would go to bed for a while and Kelly would entertain them.

Having company helped a great deal. We tried to invite someone every weekend so that we would have something to look forward to and feel like we had some semblance of a social life. Trying to maintain a social life and positive attitude is difficult, yet crucial.

Most of our friends accepted our invitations, but a few were too uncomfortable and chose not to. While their behavior was hurtful, those experiences reinforced a greater appreciation for the people who were supportive.

While I was pregnant with Colin, our need for support was much greater. I don't know what we would have done without the assistance of our families. My 11 weeks in the hospital seemed like an eternity and I came to depend on the consistent visits I received from certain family members.

Because we had moved from our home, I contacted friends to let them know where Kelly and Will were living and that I was hospitalized for the duration of my pregnancy. The reactions I received were varied and often surprising. I had a couple of friends who faithfully visited each week. One friend occasionally brought lunch while another came weekly to enjoy long talks.

But I was saddened that many people never contacted me after finding out I was hospitalized. Friends and family members who never took the time to call, send a note, or visit during those three months caused a deep hurt. In a couple of instances it has left a rift in our relationship because I never understood why they chose to do nothing.

Every bedresting mom has her own stories of hurt, disappointment, or anger, so don't feel alone if you are having these feelings. There are many reasons why people distance themselves from difficult situations, and you may never understand why people reacted the way they did.

Be grateful for all signs of support you *do* receive and attempt to move past any hurt and disappointment.

Chapter Eight

Words Of Wisdom For Husbands

Written by Kelly McCann

I will never forget the first sign of trouble in Mary Ann's pregnancy. We had taken a trip to the North Shore of Lake Superior and I encouraged her to do some hiking in the woods. We went a little further than we had planned and strained ourselves more than we should have. I will always remember the fear I experienced when she started having pains on the way home, a fear that stayed with me for the next 22 weeks. Although I learned later that any strenuous activity would have had the same effect on Mary Ann, I nevertheless felt guilty.

The first month following that trip was stressful. I waited each day to hear about any progress she may have made and what her doctor said. It became clear after three weeks that she wasn't improving, only getting a little worse each day. I began to realize that her doctor had no intention of letting her off bedrest even though every week he said, "Let's see where you're at next week."

In the beginning of Mary Ann's bedrest, before her situation worsened, she was able to do some things around the apartment. She could go out occasionally and spend time in the living room during evening hours. We had friends over and she could visit without too much trouble. Gradually this changed and I remember when the fear and uncertainty of her situation finally hit me.

I was at my mother's house for a holiday gathering. Mary Ann was going to drive over after her appointment with the doctor. She called from the doctor's office and told me to come get her because she couldn't drive. She'd had some strong contractions on the way to the doctor and needed to pull over on the shoulder of the freeway. In addition, she began to have some strong contractions while at the office and her doctor said she needed to be driven home. As I was driving to pick her up I wondered what had happened, and how it had gotten so bad.

From that day forward our lives were held in the grip of the unknown. We trusted her doctor implicitly and followed his instructions closely. Mary Ann started taking medicine for her contractions and they seemed to ease a bit. It wasn't long before her dosage had increased several times to the point where she was taking dozens of pills a day. While we knew this could not continue, we didn't know what was next.

I began taking over the household chores as Mary Ann spent more and more time in bed. We soon fell into a rhythm of dinners in bed, watching TV, playing cards, and renting movies. I would do the grocery shopping, laundry, and cleaning. We had to be creative with meals so that Mary Ann had lunches prepared for her from the night before.

As the weeks passed, Mary Ann's bedrest became monotonous and she'd spend many hours a day cross-stitching, monitoring contractions, and watching TV. She was often awake until 2:00 a.m. or later with bad contractions. The boredom affected me, too, as we no longer went out, visited anyone, or were able to be physically intimate. I became more and more frustrated with my powerlessness.

Changing Expectations

I knew from working in social services that we were dealing with our daily lives in a similar way to someone who has a chronic illness or disability. The only difference was that we knew there was an end to the disability and we hoped it would lead to a healthy baby. But knowing the end did not make our daily routine any easier. The dark cloud of fear hung heavy over us and we each prayed in our own way for a healthy baby.

I began a daily prayer that asked God to place a circle of love and protection around Mary Ann and the baby.

I also began to take life one day at a time and was grateful for each week of progress toward the baby's viability. I learned that when I was powerless to change the situation I needed to turn to God to help carry the fear, pain, and anger. When I started to trust more and feel at ease, I was better able to deal with my feelings. People often asked me how I survived each day. I would reply that I just went through my days taking everything as it came, doing what needed to be done.

With regard to expectations, Mary Ann's first pregnancy was the most difficult for me. We had only been married five months when her bedrest started, so many of our plans and desires had to be put on hold. We had wanted to develop friendships and go out and socialize but we couldn't because of the pregnancy. The benefit was that we became closer friends and spent a lot more time hanging out together.

One of the biggest challenges we faced was having a conversation. It seemed that Mary Ann could never finish a sentence without being stopped by a contraction. We had always enjoyed long talks, but suddenly our conversations were continually being interrupted. Talk a little, wait for the contraction to pass, and then talk some more. We didn't have a normal conversation again until after the baby was born. While it may seem like a small thing, it was a quality of life issue for me.

When The Going Gets Tough

As the other person in this relationship, you have the most flexibility in how you respond to your partner's bedrest. She is both physically limited and limited by her doctor's orders. You, however, have the ability make things better for both of you and can even turn this challenging time into an opportunity to learn. Most importantly, you can make life a little easier for her.

Your partner needs you now – probably more than she is willing to admit – and you have an opportunity to make things better for her and the baby. Start with the little things: give her a backrub, make her some hot chocolate, or offer to go to the video store. Ask her if she needs anything. The simple fact that you are thinking about her well-being will cheer her up.

Work shorter days if you can. There are a thousand reasons why you can't, but try to make it work. There may not be a time when your family's needs are this important. When you are not there, your wife is dealing with this alone. Call her on your lunch hour. Share a story. If she has a computer, send her e-mail. Keep in touch. Bring her flowers or a special gift when you know it has been an especially rough day.

Find things to do with your wife that create connectedness, like playing a board or card game.

We played a lot of Scrabble, Gin Rummy, Trivial Pursuit, and Cribbage.

I also would find new solitaire games for Mary Ann to play. She found some of them addictive and they helped to pass the time.

Get to know the baby. Talk to the baby and feel it moving and kicking.

Both of our children were very busy in-utero, moving and kicking all the time. It became humorous when I would tell William to settle down and it seemed the tone of my voice helped him go to sleep. It felt good to know that the boys were familiar with both our voices when they were born.

Try to go to all of the doctor's appointments, if possible.

Doctor appointments were special times for us. I enjoyed being able to see the baby grow on the ultrasound each week and share in the discussion with the doctor about Mary Ann's progress. We also enjoyed the time we had together outside of the house, often going out to lunch after the appointment. Those times gave us some semblance of a normal life because we weren't able to go out any other time. It was a little thing, but it sure felt good to be out of the house with Mary Ann.

Provide encouragement whenever you can. Try to understand your wife's pain and discomfort. Let her know how much you love and respect her for what she is doing for you and the baby. Be there when she needs someone to talk to or a shoulder to cry on. Bedrest is a painful experience both physically and emotionally, so be mindful of that when she seems hard to live with. While you can never really feel what she feels, she can feel your acceptance, encouragement, and unconditional love.

Taking Care Of Yourself

It is not good to burn your candle at both ends for too long. You need to learn how to take care of yourself while you are taking care of everyone else. I tried to do something fun for myself everyday. Sometimes I would spend time reading, or working/playing on the computer.

When Mary Ann was on bedrest with William I spent a lot of time on the computer. The internet was just getting started and it was cool to be accessing computers in Russia and Japan. It was a good outlet for me – something new to learn and re-energize me.

If you like to exercise, go for a run or a workout at the gym. Play some pick-up basketball, go golfing, or anything else that interests you. It is important for you to enjoy something that takes you away from your worries and concerns. Encourage your wife to do the same. If she can find something enjoyable to do which can distract her for a little while, she will be happier.

Reaching Out To Others

It is important to tell others what is going on in your life. Tell your boss that you will need a more flexible schedule, or inquire about the possibility of working from home for an hour or two each day. Tell your co-workers what is happening. My co-workers were always willing to cover for me if I needed to go to a doctor's appointment or be at home for awhile.

Your extended family can also be a great source of moral and emotional support. When Mary Ann was in the hospital our families helped us by watching William when I was working or at the hospital. It is often difficult to ask family or friends for help, but if you make an effort to share your burden, the results may be surprising.

Preparing For The Baby

Start shopping for the baby when you feel ready. I don't think I shopped before either of my boys reached 28 weeks gestation. After we reached that milestone we knew there was a better chance they would survive an early birth and I had a little less fear of miscarriage or stillbirth.

It was a powerful moment for me when I went to the Carter's store and bought some newborn layette clothing for William. I felt the excitement of impending fatherhood and started to realize what that meant. I'd spent so much time focused on the pregnancy itself that I had pushed aside the other more natural feelings, like excitement and fear of being a father for the first time.

I had a tendency to become so focused on the day-to-day struggles of life with pregnancy bedrest that I was not able go through the typical experiences associated with pregnancy. We didn't go to childbirth classes, have a baby shower, go shopping together, or decorate the nursery. These were all losses that were hard to accept – I had waited for 30 years to be a father and felt I missed out on so much.

One positive result of this preoccupation with the pregnancy was that the baby's birth was a relief, and the normal impact a newborn has on a family was somewhat minimized. While we did go through an adjustment period of having a new person affecting the household, we felt that each of our children had already been having an impact for months before they were born. We already knew how to incorporate them into our family and waking up in the night was easier than living with the fears endured during pregnancy.

Life In The Hospital

Hospitalization is stressful for everyone in the family. The physical separation greatly impacts your relationship with your wife and the surroundings do little to foster a homey atmosphere. Most hospitals are starting to realize the impact that long-term hospitalization has on families and are trying to make changes. Long-term parking passes, movie-lending libraries, and extended visiting hours were all helpful. Bringing pictures and wall hangings from home seemed to help Mary Ann a great deal.

If you are going to be visiting a lot or staying for long periods, bring something for yourself, such as a book, that you only read while at the hospital. Having something of your own in the room will help you feel more at home.

Nurses

It is important for you to get to know the nurses. You will learn quickly which ones are tuned into your needs as husband and wife. They will try to be unobtrusive and willing to leave you alone for longer periods of time. There were a few times when they helped us have a romantic dinner or let us use their freezer for some of Mary Ann's favorite ice cream.

The nurses are also a good source of information about your wife's condition and emotional well-being. They are knowledgeable about hospital policies regarding parking and visitation – it took me three weeks to realize I could park for free, rather than hourly, simply because I had not asked.

Meals And Special Treats

I would often check in with Mary Ann during the day to find out what the hospital's menu selections were like. If they were particularly bad, or she didn't get what was ordered for lunch or dinner, I would bring her dinner or dessert.

I also tried to bring special surprises to cheer her up. It is important to try and stay as close as possible, and little gifts help show her that you are thinking about her.

Other Children

Mary Ann was hospitalized with Colin when Will was 2½. I brought William to visit about every other day and we'd usually stay for about an hour. Our ritual included going to McDonalds either before or after our visit.

Not caring for William was one of the most distressing situations Mary Ann had to face while hospitalized, and William's visits helped them both. While he did not understand everything that was going on, William did know why his mommy was in the hospital, that she loved him and he was still her little boy. William grew up a lot that summer as different family members helped raise him. He enjoyed going to the different houses and playing with his cousins.

Life After Bedrest

I wondered if our life would ever return to normal after bedrest because we changed in so many ways during the experience. We learned new ways of dealing with stress and found new reserves of strength we didn't know we had. Reality changes with a difficult pregnancy. Previously unknown experiences like contractions, subcutaneous terbutaline pumps, administering Betamethasone shots, and weekly visits to the doctor became routine parts of life.

I will never look at my children without a full appreciation of the gift of life they are. With William and Colin, I experience all the joys of growing, learning, and exploring a wonderful new world – a world that helped bring Colin and William home to us.

The miracle of their births has fostered a new closeness between Mary Ann and me. The forced separation of hospital bedrest helped us become more independent while also showing us how interdependent we are. We endured a great hardship in our marriage and we grew as a couple because of it. We have a strong appreciation for the gift of life and do not take it for granted. We thank God everyday for giving us healthy children.

It took several months for us to get back into a pattern of life together. We needed to re-establish duties and roles around the house. We needed to share more of the childcare and discipline. But most importantly, we needed to relate to each other as we had before each bedrest pregnancy. We had to learn how we each had changed from the experiences and then turn that knowledge into a greater love for each other.

The psychological trauma of bedrest may remain for a long time. There are often lingering feelings of fear or disorientation. After living so close to the helplessness of a difficult pregnancy, it can take some time for those feelings to heal. This often happens as the Baby Blues or a letdown after any pregnancy, but with a bedrest pregnancy it may have other dimensions to it. Mary Ann discusses her battle with postpartum depression in Chapter 9. If you suspect that your wife may be severely depressed, you may find some of the information there to be helpful.

The psychological after-effect will be present for both you and your partner. For months afterward, you may find yourself unconsciously waiting for her to stop what she is doing and hold her stomach as she has a contraction.

I am not thankful for the pain Mary Ann and I had to go through, but it was a unique learning experience for us both, and I know I would go through it again to experience the joys of fatherhood. While I chose to accept the struggles and challenges we faced, I was often bitter and angry, and wondered "why us?" I never understood why it had to be so difficult, but I also I knew that resentment and anger would not help me, my wife, or my son.

I am thankful for the growth in myself and in my marriage that the bedrest experience offered. Because of it I feel more confident when facing challenges and more secure in the knowledge that Mary Ann and I can deal with anything we may encounter.

Chapter Nine

After Your Baby Arrives...Life After Bedrest

I f you have not yet delivered your baby, I recommend that you postpone reading this chapter until your baby is born.

Congratulations on the birth of your baby! You have much to be proud of and grateful for. Your body has just endured a very long battle and it is normal if you are feeling tired. After bedrest, however, there are often unexpected physical and emotional issues to cope with. This chapter is intended to help you through the myriad of changes in your life and assure you that many of your feelings are completely normal. It is not intended to serve as a substitute for appropriate medical advice, and, in fact, it is my hope that you will consider seeking medical attention for any postpartum difficulties.

Physical Symptoms Associated With the Postpartum Stage

Fatigue

Every woman experiences fatigue following the birth of a baby. This is the most common symptom of postpartum recovery. Your body needs time to recuperate from the trauma and stresses of giving birth. The demands of a new infant are also intense and time-consuming, often resulting in lack of sleep. If your baby was premature, you are probably sleeping even less, since many preemies are up to feed as often as every 90 minutes.

During this time, it is essential that you take care of yourself.

Napping when your baby naps will do wonders for your energy level. The laundry can wait. House cleaning can wait. And eating frozen foods or ordering a pizza can minimize dinner preparations. Allow your partner to share some of the responsibilities for caring for the baby and the housework – after all, he has already been doing some of this while you were on bedrest.

If this is your first baby, it is perfectly normal to feel completely overwhelmed. Concentrate your energies on learning how to care for your new baby and yourself. For women on bedrest, fatigue is an even greater issue, since your body was inactive for so long. Don't be surprised if you are exhausted after your first trip to the grocery store. It will get better, but it's a long, slow process of recovery. Each day you will become a little stronger and start to feel more energetic...just give it time.

If you have friends and relatives who offer assistance...accept it. Many people offer to bring a meal or help with caring for the baby. Don't be afraid to say "yes."

Vaginal Tear/Hemorrhoids/Uteran Discomfort

Delivering a baby is, for most women, a physically demanding experience. If you delivered vaginally and your doctor performed an episiotomy, or if you suffered a vaginal tear, you will need time to heal. It is important for you to follow all of your doctor's orders and suggestions. Nurses will also have some suggestions to help you feel more comfortable, so seek their advice.

Warm baths are soothing and offer relaxation from the new stresses and worries of motherhood. Sitting on a donut pillow (an inflated pillow with a hole in the middle) can also ease some of the discomfort while sitting. Hemorrhoids are often a problem after delivery. Do not hesitate to ask your nurse or doctor for some external ointment to ease the pain. They may suggest that you take a stool softener for a few days to minimize the pain and pressure.

If you delivered by Caesarean section, you will probably experience pain while your uterus and abdomen heal. The recovery after a C-section is a bit longer and you will most likely stay in the hospital for three or four days. You may be offered medications for pain relief and you have the right to decide whether you wish to take them. If you are breastfeeding, it is important to ask which medications are safe to take.

After you are released from the hospital, it is important to rest and follow your doctor's orders. Giving birth is hard work, and if you have been on bedrest, you will need to give your body extra time to heal. My own experiences lead me to believe that the physical discomfort of the postpartum period is exacerbated by the amount of time you were in bed prior to delivery. Just keep reminding yourself that each day will bring added strength and less discomfort.

If you were on complete bedrest for more than a few weeks, you may discover some other physical problems following delivery of your baby. I urge you to seek medical attention if you are at all concerned about these or any other issues.

Back Pain

It is not uncommon to experience backaches while pregnant. However, if you continue to experience back pain after you deliver, consider consulting a physician. Bedrest often results in back pain that will not be alleviated by delivery. Lying on one side, often using your arm to prop your head, can cause significant stress to the muscles in your neck, shoulders and back. The longer you were on bedrest, the more severe your back problems may be.

I suffered from neck and back problems after both of my bedrest pregnancies. After being up and moving around again I experienced pain much of the time. While I benefited greatly from chiropractic care, I required treatments three times a week for several months before being able to return to household tasks without pain.

I worried that my back problems would return when I was put on modified bedrest 10 weeks into my second pregnancy. So, when I was put on complete bedrest shortly thereafter, I knew I needed to receive help. My consultations with a chiropractor who had experience treating pregnancy related back problems helped a great deal.

(Important: Consult with your OB/GYN to ask if chiropractic treatments are appropriate and safe for you.)

After I delivered and returned home, my back once again hurt most of the time. The 11 weeks I spent lying on my left side in a hospital bed caused constant neck, shoulder, and lower back pain. I knew that losing the 50 pounds I had gained would alleviate a lot of my pain, but I felt I needed medical attention. It was crucial for my chiropractor to understand the extent of my bedrest and the position I was usually in while in bed.

I also had intense pains in my hips that neither my OB/GYN nor the chiropractor could diagnose. After several months the discomfort had not dissipated and I was unable to run up stairs without a throbbing pain in my hips. I consulted with an Orthopedic Specialist who determined I had bursitis, which is an inflammation of the cavity surrounding the hip joint. Bursitis is common among individuals who are bedridden for long periods of time and can occur in any joint in the body. Several weeks of ultrasound treatments and a few cortisone injections helped a great deal. I wish that I had known that this pain was treatable because I spent several months waiting for the problem to remedy itself.

Foot Problems

This may sound crazy, but believe me, it's not. After spending three months in a hospital bed where I was always too warm to even wear socks, putting shoes back on was less than enjoyable. I couldn't understand why I was getting blisters. My shoes were not new, yet after several hours in even comfortable sneakers, my feet ached, and blisters covered my toes.

My feet were simply not accustomed to wearing shoes. They grew a half size during my pregnancy, so the first thing I needed to do was buy a new pair of comfortable shoes. I wore shoes for shorter periods of time to allow my feet time to reacclimate, but it took a couple of months before I was comfortable again.

If you have more serious problems with your feet, do not hesitate to consult with a podiatrist. Feet often grow during pregnancy, prolonged illness, or other times when shoes aren't worn for long periods of time. Corns, blisters, and aching feet are all common problems for women who have been on bedrest.

As tempted as you might be to postpone a visit to the dentist, you would be wise to make an appointment soon after your baby is born. If you do require dental work, the sooner you are able to complete it, the less painful it will be.

While I was in the hospital, I was somewhat tentative about thoroughly brushing and flossing my teeth because my gums bled. While many pregnant women experience bleeding gums, being on Magnesium Sulfate often exacerbates the problem.

Emotional / Psychological Adjustments

If this is your first baby, you may feel as if you are on an emotional roller coaster. The adjustment to parenthood can be overwhelming. In addition, the hormone levels in your body need time to level out.

If this is not your first baby, you are most likely aware of the emotional highs and lows experienced following a birth. For most women the joy and excitement overshadow any sort of anxiety or depression. But many women experience mild depression, often referred to as baby blues, soon after delivery. In fact, 50-75% of all new mothers experience some blues, often related to hormonal imbalances. Some women attribute their varying emotions to a lack of sleep, but there are many reasons why you, as a new mom just coming off bedrest, may be feeling depressed:

- A prolonged hospitalization for you;
- A prolonged hospitalization for your baby;
- Feeling a sense of disappointment about your delivery (many women who require a Cesarean birth feel a sense of loss about not having delivered vaginally);
- Sudden overwhelming feelings of inadequacy about your abilities as a mother;
- Changes in your postpartum body. Many bedresting moms gain more than the average 25-30 pounds and feel frustrated about their body size after delivery;
- A sense of loss at no longer being pregnant and feeling that intense physical and emotional connection to your baby;

- Feeling emotionally and physically distant from your partner due to the demands of your new baby, your level of fatigue, and your need to continue to refrain from sexual intercourse.

Any of these issues can cause postpartum baby blues. For most women these feelings do not last more than a few weeks. There are good days and bad days, and the bad days are often accentuated by your baby's temperament.

The support and understanding of your partner is essential during this time. It is important for you to realize that your partner is also adjusting to parenthood and the changes in your relationship. Open, honest communication is necessary for you both. Talk about your fears and apprehensions and offer each other support and encouragement.

If you were on bedrest for more than a few weeks your baby blues may not dissipate as quickly as for some. If you delivered a premature baby, you may find yourself tired most of the time, especially if you are feeding every two hours. You probably feel like you spend all of your time caring for your new baby, and housework, laundry, cooking, grocery shopping, caring for other children, and making time for your partner are too overwhelming to even think about.

If this describes how you are feeling, I can honestly tell you that I have been there. I know those feelings because I lived it.

My Experience With Postpartum Depression

After my first son was born I experienced the baby blues. I was exhausted and weak and had little energy for anything other than caring for him. I remember the first time I went grocery shopping after he was born. I was so excited to get out by myself and feel a sense of freedom that bedrest had robbed from me. I returned from the grocery store so tired I had to take a nap. I found it extremely frustrating and depressing that I didn't have my old energy back.

Once I learned to take care of myself and not expect too much too soon, I was able to recover more quickly. I tried to relax while acknowledging that caring for my son was a full-time job. I rested while the baby napped and went for walks or did something for myself when Kelly was able to relieve me.

After my second son was born, my exhaustion was more severe. Colin had to be awakened every two hours to feed and Kelly was working a second job, which meant that I was alone four nights a week. The first three or four months of Colin's life are a bit of a blur. When I wasn't caring for Colin, I was trying to re-establish my relationship with William. My pregnancy had greatly altered our mother-son relationship. William spent two months in daycare, evenings with his dad so I could stay in bed, then three months living at his grandma's and cared for by relatives while I was hospitalized. It took us a long time to re-establish our relationship.

I knew that fatigue and depression were normal, so I kept telling myself that it would improve. And, as always, whenever someone asked me how I was, I told him or her that everything was great. I never told anyone that I felt like I was slipping further into depression.

As Colin approached five months, I felt that life was settling down a bit. He was sleeping better and past much of his initial colic and irritability.

I kept waiting to feel better, but it seemed like I was living behind a dark cloud. My life was everything that I had always hoped it would be – I had a wonderfully supportive husband, the children I had dreamed of and prayed for, I was home full-time like I wanted to be – yet, I was always sad.

I cried, often uncontrollably, at least once a day. I was withdrawn from Kelly and he couldn't understand why. I had no interest in spending time with other people, and when I did have plans, I often made up excuses to avoid going out. I was too embarrassed to admit this to anyone. I kept waiting for these terrible feelings to go away, but they never did. I felt that I was slowly losing my marriage and the family that I had worked so hard to have. Kelly tried to reach out, but I continued to push him away.

When I finally realized the detrimental effect it was having on my marriage, I knew that I had to get help. I called one of the nurses at my OB/GYN's office that I felt comfortable talking to. I was almost too embarrassed and scared to even talk to her. When she started asking me questions about my moods and feelings, I heard myself answering "yes" to each one. I broke down, sobbing, because I truly believed that I was going crazy. She told me that she felt I was suffering from postpartum depression. She explained that, unlike the baby blues, postpartum depression (often referred to as PPD) does not go away within a few weeks after delivery. It can last for several months and requires medical attention. I immediately made an appointment to see my doctor.

Understanding Postpartum Depression

At least 10-20% of all new mothers will experience some form of PPD. Many researchers believe that this percentage is higher among women who have experienced a high-risk pregnancy, prolonged bedrest, and/or premature birth. There are many symptoms of PPD with variations in the severity of the symptoms. These symptoms may include, but are not limited to:

- Fatigue and exhaustion
- A pervasive feeling of sadness, depression, loneliness, or hopelessness
- Appetite and sleep disturbances
- Poor concentration and confusion
- Memory loss, including short-term memory loss
- Overconcern for the baby
- Uncontrollable crying
- Irritability
- Lack of interest in the baby
- Guilt, inadequacy, worthlessness
- Fear of harming the baby
- Fear of harming yourself
- Exaggerated highs and/or lows
- Decreased/lack of interest in sex

If you are experiencing any of these symptoms, I would urge you to seek medical attention. Your OB/GYN should be familiar with your symptoms and able to determine if you are suffering from PPD. If you are apprehensive about talking with your doctor (a common concern), consider talking first with one of the nurses or nurse practitioners you have a good relationship with. Or, if you prefer, contact one of the support agencies listed in Chapter 11, and ask for a referral to a psychiatrist or psychologist in your area that specializes in PPD.

There are several possible treatments for PPD, including, but not limited to: prescription medications such as an anti-depressant, lifestyle changes or alterations, participation in a PPD support group (usually sponsored by your local hospital), and counseling from a therapist who specializes in PPD.

In the Appendix at the end of this book are some further resources. Depression After Delivery (DAD) offers women and their partners information about PPD in addition to a thorough listing, by state, of professional therapists who are trained to work with women suffering from it. DAD also has a network of volunteers who have all dealt with PPD, and are willing to be matched with women to offer them support. Even if you are already working with your OB/GYN, I encourage you to contact DAD. They will be happy to send you additional information.

I was treated with an anti-depressant, Zoloft, for over a year, which is the average length of time women are treated with medications. I was amazed at the improvement in my feelings and outlook. The Zoloft saved me and helped restore my marriage and family life. I also began truly processing, on my own, how my bedrest experiences had impacted and changed me. I began writing and journaling, as a way to understand my feelings, a crucial step to moving on. My chapter about the losses associated with bedrest pregnancies is a result of my journal. I needed to mourn those many losses, accept them, and then move forward. My sadness and depression hindered and weighed me down.

I still feel twinges of sadness, particularly when I see pregnant women who are able to have normal pregnancies. I never shopped for my babies' layettes, attended childbirth classes, shared the joys and challenges of physical intimacy with my husband while being pregnant, or entertained thoughts of having additional children. These losses are painful, but they taught us and brought us together in a unique way. We are stronger, individually and as a couple, for having these experiences.

Do not hesitate to get help if you need it. I suffered for too long being afraid to tell anyone how I was feeling. I was sure that people would think I was weak or unable to cope with my two children. I had no idea how common PPD is, or how serious it can be if left untreated. Open up to your partner and share your feelings, concerns, and fears. If you are suffering from PPD, your partner and family already know that something is wrong. While you may think you are hiding it from them, you're not.

Chapter Ten

Deciding About Another Pregnancy

F or many couples who have lived through the physical, mental, and emotional ordeal of a high-risk pregnancy, deciding about future pregnancies can be stressful. A child brings great joy and the difficult memories of bedrest tend to fade as you stare into the eyes of your beautiful baby. The decision whether to have another child is ultimately one that only you and your partner can make. Obviously the decision is easy if your bedrest pregnancy was the last, and/or only, child that you both wanted. However, if your bedrest pregnancy was your first, or you fully intended to have more children, you may be nervous about the future.

The first thing you should do is have an open discussion with your OB/GYN about your bedrest pregnancy and how it may affect future pregnancies. If you have a pre-existing medical condition or disability such as diabetes, epilepsy, lupus, or hypertension, your chances of encountering problems in the future may be quite high. A congenital malformation of the uterus, or an incompetent cervix, also puts you at high risk. While you may already know your risk is high, you might not realize the extent of the problems you are likely to face. You and your partner need to make a decision based on sound medical advice, which is why a serious discussion with your physician is imperative.

As noted in Chapter 1, Kelly and I were not surprised that my second pregnancy was worse than my first. We were told this would most likely be the case and warned that extensive hospitalization was a possibility.

If your bedrest was due to a multiple pregnancy, your doctor will probably tell you that future complications are unlikely. In fact, your chances of having another multiple pregnancy are quite low, although increased if you are using fertility drugs.

If you are among the thousands of women who had a bedrest pregnancy that could not be readily explained, your doctor may tell you that your risk of complications in the future is relatively low. Placental abruption, placenta previa, premature rupture of the membranes (the bag of waters) and, sometimes, premature labor, are often confined to one pregnancy. You should not assume that you would have the same problem(s) again. However, you should also not assume that you are free of any risks. Your doctor can help you understand what may have caused the problems in the bedrest pregnancy and explain the risks for the future.

You and your partner should realize that if your doctor does not offer an explanation for your complications, it could mean the problem is difficult to diagnose. Kelly and I were originally told that the complications I suffered with my first pregnancy were not likely to repeat. I had a placental abruption, and then, several weeks later, began premature labor. My doctor thought that the premature labor was directly related to the placental abruption, as is usually the case. He told us there was a chance I could have problems again, but it was not a certainty. It was only because of some infertility testing that a congenital malformation of my uterus was discovered and explained why I had such a hard time. The placental abruption and premature labor were directly related to my bicornet uterus. We were amazed this problem was not found on the countless ultrasounds I had.

While it is important to understand that there are never any guarantees, seeking medical advice and conducting your own research will enable you to make a more informed decision about another pregnancy.

I was surprised by the number of people who asked me how my husband and I were able to make the decision to have a second child, particularly after we were told how difficult a subsequent pregnancy would be. It felt like people were judging our decision, especially once we had difficulties even becoming pregnant. The comments hurt, particularly since most of the people challenging us already had the families they wanted. It may sound crazy, but Kelly's and my desire for a second child was stronger than for our first. Our desire to have our first child was balanced with a fear of the unknown, but after our son was born, the joys of life as a parent were much greater than either of us ever anticipated.

We decided we wanted to give William a sibling, and in fact, had always intended to have more than two children. We never lost sight of that goal, although I often contemplated the irony of our decision. Because I spent the summer in a hospital bed, I missed an entire summer with William in order to give him someone to share the rest of his summers with.

Many couples struggle with the decision to have another child if they know the pregnancy is high-risk. I know that if Kelly had not been 100% supportive, it could have been detrimental to the future of our marriage and family. The decision about another high-risk pregnancy should never be made on your own. Some women decide they will never contemplate another pregnancy because any risk of bedrest is too much. I have spoken with women who refuse to discuss another pregnancy even though their husbands would like to have another child. For these women the pressures are often great. One woman told me that the biggest obstacle for her and her husband was that this issue could not be solved through compromise.

Another important consideration is the life of any future child. If you delivered a premature baby, you most likely already know the fear and worry of your child's first hours, days, or weeks. For many couples who have watched their child spend several weeks in a Neonatal ICU, the experience is one they do not wish to repeat. For them, any risk of premature delivery, or of having a disabled child, is too great. Some of these parents consider adoption as an option. Naturally, a high-risk pregnancy does not mean that you will deliver prematurely, but this is an important issue for you and your partner to discuss with your OB/GYN.

For Kelly and me, one of the greatest factors in our decision to not have a third child was our concern for the health of the baby. While I would have gladly endured another pregnancy, I could not knowingly put the baby at risk. Our second child was at more risk than our first, and we knew that the next child would be at even greater risk. Every individual has their own tolerance level of what they feel they can endure, and, as a couple, we had reached our threshold for the amount of risk we were willing to live with in order to have another child.

Questions To Consider

If you decide you want to try and get pregnant again, and you are relatively certain that you will be put on bedrest, there are a few factors to consider. You and your partner may wish to discuss the following subjects, and try to make some decisions now. For example:

Your Children

How old would you like your child(ren) to be before you become pregnant again? You may wish to wait until your children are able to understand your situation or participate in small household tasks. If you are an at-home mother, will you need to arrange for childcare if you are on bedrest?

Finances

How will another bedrest pregnancy affect your family's finances? If you are working outside of the home, how will you be able to adjust to a modified, or full, loss of your income? If you are at home, how will you be able to adjust to the cost of daycare or a nanny for your child(ren)?

Health Insurance

If you are responsible for a percentage of your maternity, and/or postnatal medical expenses, how might that affect your financial situation? Are you anticipating a change in your health insurance in the next year?

Support

Are family and friends available to help you with your children and/or your home? Would it be helpful to try to plan a pregnancy to coordinate with the care your child(ren) may need? (i.e. Do you have a sibling or close friend who is already expecting? What time of year is best for your children?)

Job

Are you anticipating a job change for either you or your partner? This may reduce the amount of available sick/vacation leave. It may also change your health insurance.

Moving From Your Home

Are you contemplating a move from your home in the next year?

Family Life

How will another bedrest pregnancy affect your child(ren)? What concerns or fears do you have about the affects on your family?

If you and your partner decide that your family is complete, the decision may sometimes be hard to accept. Kelly and I have never doubted that we made the right decision. My doctor gave us straightforward medical advice and we knew that a third pregnancy was dangerous for the baby and me. And, the thought of enduring infertility a second time was not something we wanted to think about. Although we are certain our decision was the correct the one, we both have moments when we wonder what it would have been like to have more children.

Chapter Eleven

Resources For Bedrest Moms

Clothing, Baby Products, Furniture, Toys, And Equipment

The companies in this section offer maternity and baby/layette clothing, as well as baby accessories, supplies, furniture, toys, and equipment for both breastfeeding and bottle feeding.

Some companies offer toll-free numbers that you can call to request a catalog. For those of you with access to the Internet, I have included web pages and some e-mail addresses. Many companies now have complete web catalogs for on-line shopping.

Abracadabra Maternity

www.momshop.com

• Full selection of maternity clothes that are available for on-line purchase.

Baby Catalog

www.babycatalog.com

A web site devoted to the on-line purchase of furniture, bedding, books, toys, and nursery supplies.

The Baby Depot

www.coat.com

Also known as Burlington Coat Factory, The Baby Depot is an on-line shopping service.

Baby & You (JCPenney)

800-222-6161

www.shopping.jcpenney.com

• Maternity clothes, layette and baby clothing, furniture, and some nursery accessories. All available for on-line purchase.

Century Products Company

800-837-4044

• Car seats, strollers, etc.

The Company Store
800-323-8000
www.thecompanystore.com
- Clothing and linens.

Daisy Kingdom
503-222-9033
- Nursery ensembles, which are available in do-it-yourself kits or ready-made ensembles.

The Gymboree Corporation
700 Airport Blvd. Suite #200
Burlingame, CA 94010
www.gymboree.com
e-mail: giftcenter@gymmail.com
- On-line store for purchasing baby clothes. Also, information about the Gymboree infant classes.

Internet Baby
www.internetbaby.com
This is advertised as the "largest on-line shopping service" available to new parents. They offer feeding supplies, safety products, clothing, toys, nursery furniture and supplies, and diapering products.

Le Petite Baby
12105 Leeward Walk Circle
Alpharetta GA 30202
770-475-3247
www.no-odor.com/preemie
e-mail: lepetite@no-odor.com
- This company is the world's largest supplier of clothing for premature (weighing less than seven pounds) infants. Their on-line store allows for purchase of clothing.

Maternity Fashions & Little Ones
739 Brookwood Village
Birmingham AL 35209
800-290-8910
www.maternityfashions.com
e-mail: fashions@quicklink.net
- On-line purchase of maternity clothes, layette/baby clothes, and some furniture and baby accessories.

Medela Rental Services
800-836-5968
www.medela.com
- Breast-pump rentals. Web-page offers information and on-line lactation consultants to answer questions.

Mother's Nature
703 Main Street
Watertown CT 06795
888-875-4647
www.babyholder.com
- On-line shopping available. This company offers cloth diapers, nursing clothes, baby slings and carriers, and more.

One Step Ahead
P.O. Box 517
Lake Bluff IL 60044
800-274-8440
- Infant feeding and diapering products, toys, furniture, and baby-proofing/safety products.

The Online Preemie Store
508-378-7142
www.preemiestore.com
- Preemie products, resources, and a discussion forum.

The Preemie Store
17195 Newhope Street
Suite 105
Fountain Valley CA 92708
800-676-TINY
www.preemie.com
• Another company that specializes in
  clothing for premature infants. Many
  of their products are specifically
  designed for use in the Neonatal
  Intensive Care Unit.

The Right Start Catalog
800-548-8531
• Toys, nursery aids, feeding products.

Seventh Generation
800-456-1177
• Organic and natural baby products.

Spencer's
238 Willow Street
Post Office Box #988
Mount Airy NC 27030
800-633-9111
www.spencers.com
e-mail: custserv@spencers.com
• Spencer's is a company well-known
  for layette and infant clothing. They
  have a well-organized web page,
  complete with on-line shopping
  services. They also have a catalog
  you can request.

Wal-Mart
www.wal-mart.com
Wal-Mart offers a complete on-line
store. Their entire store is available,
just click on the "Infant and Baby" icon
to move to that section.

Whole Nine Months
3545 Midway Drive
San Diego CA 92110
619-274-0784
www.wholenine.com
• Maternity clothes and nursing tops
  available for on-line purchase.

Consumer Information

The following is a listing of consumer information hotlines of some of the larger manufacturers of infant and baby furniture and equipment including car seats, strollers, playpens, and toys. When known, I have included information about what type of consumer services are available.

Century Products Corporation
800-837-4044
• Call for a catalog of products and a listing of stores in your area which carry many Century products. Credit card orders are also accepted.

Cosco Consumer Relations
800-544-1108
www.coscoinc.com
• Catalog available for purchasing car seats, strollers, cribs, high chairs, etc. Web page includes detailed information and photos of the many products offered, as well as a "Where To Shop" guide.

Evenflo Consumer Affairs
800-356-2229
www.evenflo.com
• Feeding products and baby accessories. While there is not a catalog available, there are brochures available that describe their products. The web page offers full product information and photos.

Fisher Price
800-432-5437
www.fisherprice.com
• "Toy Fare" catalog available for $5. Catalog includes all Fisher Price toys, clothing, baby monitors, and other products.

Gerber Baby Products
800-443-7237
www.gerber.com
• There is not a catalog available, but there are brochures and informational packets which are available. This phone number is staffed 24 hours/day. There is also a mailing list to receive coupon packets and information about their baby foods, infant formula, and feeding products. The web page is comprehensive and allows consumers an opportunity to ask questions of the Gerber Product Specialists.

Johnson & Johnson
Consumer Products Information
800-526-3967
www.jnj.com
• Johnson & Johnson does not have a catalog, nor do they accept direct customer orders. However, they have product information packets and a mailing list.

Proctor & Gamble
800-582-2623
• One of the few manufacturers of preemie diapers; sold by cases containing 240 diapers. Credit card telephone orders accepted.

Web Sites For Parents Of Preemies

America Online's Mailing List Directory: www.idot.aol.com

Babycenter.com: www.babycenter.com

Classic Neonatology: www.csmc.edu/neonatology/classics.html

Parenting bulletin boards and chat rooms: www.parentsplace.com

www.familyboards.disney.com/boards

Babyhood's preemie page: www.babyhood.com/links/health/preemie

The Babies Planet Preemie site: www.thebabiesplanet.com/bbpropr.shtml

National Organizations And Support Services

American Association for Marriage and Family Therapy
1100 Seventeenth Street Northwest
Washington D.C. 20036-4601
- Provides referral information about certified Marriage and Family Therapists in your area.

American Association of Premature Infants
P.O. Box 6920
Cincinnati OH 45206
513-956-4331
www.aapi-online.org
- A non-profit advocacy organization dedicated to improving the quality of health, developmental and educational services for premature infants, children, and their families.

American Psychiatric Association
1400 K Street Northwest
Washington D.C. 20005
202-682-6000
www.psych.org
- Provides referral information about Licensed Psychiatrists in your area. Specify the area of expertise that you may need, i.e., Postpartum Depression.

American Psychological Association
750 First Street Northeast
Washington D.C. 20002-4242
800-374-2721
www.apa.org
e-mail: apacollege@apa.org

American College of Obstetrics and Gynecologists
409 12th Street Southwest
Washington D.C. 20024
202-638-5577
- Provides referrals to licensed OB/GYN clinics in your area. The ACOG will also provide you with referrals of OB/GYN's who have experience with high-risk pregnancies.

Association for the Care of Children's Health
7910 Woodmont Avenue • Suite 300
Bethesda MD 20814
800-808-ACCH
www.acch.org
- A non-profit organization dedicated to improving newborn intensive care.

The Confinement Line
c/o the Childbirth Education Association
P.O. Box 1609
Springfield VA 22151
703-941-7183
- Offers a support line and newsletter for women on bedrest. They also offer assistance to individuals seeking to start a support network in their own community.

Depression After Delivery (DAD)
P.O. Box 1282
Morrisville PA 19067
800-944-4PPD
- DAD is a non-profit organization founded for the education and support of women suffering from postpartum depression. DAD has an informational packet available at no cost. There are also telephone contacts available in many larger cities. DAD will also provide a listing of local therapists who are qualified and experienced in the area of postpartum depression.

Epilepsy Foundation of America
Landover, MD
800-332-1000
www.efa.org

High Risk Moms
P.O. Box 189165
Chicago IL 60638
708-515-5453
A support group and quarterly newsletter for those experiencing high-risk pregnancies. They also provide telephone contacts.

International Twins Association
c/o Marilyn Holmes
511 Gilpin Street
Denver CO 80209

La Leche League International

9616 Minneapolis Avenue

P.O. Box #1209

Franklin Park IL 60131

800-LaLeche

www.lalecheleague.org

- LaLeche League is an organization providing women with breastfeeding information and support. Call to find out where your local chapter is located. LaLeche League also offers support groups in major cities throughout the country. Offers a helpful web page. Women can submit questions via e-mail for answer by a qualified lactation consultant. Information is also available for women breastfeeding premature infants or multiples.

Lupus Foundation of America, Inc.

Rockville, MD

800-558-0121

www.lupus.org

- Offers free informational booklets about Lupus and pregnancy.

Mothers At Home

8310 Old Courthouse Road

Vienna VA 22183

800-783-4666

www.mah.org

e-mail: mah@mah.org

- Mothers at Home is a volunteer-based organization. They publish a monthly newsletter, Welcome Home, which contains supportive, touching, and often humorous articles written by, and for, at-home mothers. A sample newsletter is available.

National Arthritis Foundation

Atlanta, Georgia

800-283-7800

- Provides free brochures on pregnancy and arthritis. A bi-monthly magazine is also available.

National Diabetes Information and Action Line

New York City

800-DIABETES

www.diabetes.org

- Provides information and support to persons with diabetes. A booklet on diabetes and pregnancy is also available.

National Organization of Mothers of Twins Clubs, Inc.

Post Office Box #23188

Albuquerque NM 87192-1188

800-243-2276

www.nomotc.org

- A great web site offering a wealth of information about parenting twins. They oversee Twins Clubs all over the country, and the web-site will help you locate a club near you.

National Perinatal Organization

3500 East Fletcher Avenue • Suite 209

Tampa FL 33613

813-971-1008

- An association of individuals and organizations concerned with perinatal health issues. A membership-based organization that offers a quarterly newsletter.

Parents of Preemies Incorporated
P. O. Box 5183
Arlington VA 22205
301-253-6534

Parents Without Partners
8807 Colesville Road
Silver Spring MD 20910
301-588-9354

Sidelines National Support Network
P.O. Box #1808
Laguna Beach CA 92652
714-497-2265
www.sidelines.org
- This organization has many local chapters throughout the United States. The staffers of Sidelines match women on bedrest with a woman who has experienced a similar bedrest. Also available is a magazine by and for women with high-risk pregnancies.

Triplet Connection
P. O. Box 99571
Stockton CA 95209
209-474-3073
www.tripletconnection.org
- Triplet Connection is a non-profit network of caring and sharing for multiple-birth families. They provide information to families expecting triplets, quadruplets or more as well as encouragement, resources and networking opportunities for families who are parents of larger multiples.

United Way of America
701 North Fairfax Street
Alexandria VA 22314
703-836-7100
www.unitedway.org
- The United Way offers helpful programs for low income families or single parents who need assistance while on bedrest. Consult your local telephone directory for a local listing, or call their number and inquire about services and funded agencies that are available.